Wild Orphan Babies: Mammals and Birds

Wild Orphan Babies MAMMALS AND BIRDS

Caring for Them + Setting Them Free

WILLIAM J. WEBER, D.V.M.

photographs by the author

Holt Rinehart and Winston
New York

Published simultaneously in Canada by Holt, Rinehart
and Winston of Canada, Limited.

Printed in the United States of America

10 9 8 7 6 5 4 3 2 1
Second Edition

Library of Congress Cataloging in Publication Data

Weber, William J.
  Wild orphan babies.

  Bibliography: p. 152
  Includes index.
  SUMMARY: A handbook offering instruction on the
housing, feeding, and general care of orphaned wild animal
babies and how to prepare them for life in the wild.
  1.   Wildlife rescue—Juvenile literature.   2.   Wildlife
diseases—Juvenile literature.   [1.   Wildlife rescue.
2.   Wild animals as pets]   I.   Title.
QL82.2.W4   1978   639.9   78–4352
ISBN 0–03–044976–6

For my family, sons Bill and John, who help feed and care for a great many of the orphaned and injured, and helped develop the techniques we use, and for my wife Barbara, who cares for all the babies, makes formula, feeds orphans, corrected the grammar in my manuscript, and did all the typing. This is really her book.

WJW

Virtually all of us making a career of conservation, display, or control of wildlife began our careers (and our undying love for animals) with a pet squirrel, toad, snake, crow, or praying mantis. I've always felt, as a naturalist and veterinarian, that my responsibility was not to discourage this normal urge, but to direct it toward the love and respect for our natural wilderness and its inhabitants.

Dr. Don Collins
Veterinary Consultant
Topeka, Kansas

Preface

I am a veterinarian in private practice in a small city in central Florida. In 1964 my family and I moved from that city to a three-and-one-half-acre site on the shore of a clear lake. Being an Audubon member of long standing, in due course I persuaded our neighbors to join with us in having the area declared an Audubon sanctuary. Our home now occupies the center of that sanctuary.

Gradually, word of the sanctuary and our interest in wildlife spread throughout the community, and my veterinary hospital became the drop-off point for injured and orphaned wild birds and animals.

My family and I agreed to do our best to raise or heal the sick and orphaned animals and birds that were brought to us with the understanding that we would set them free when they were able to survive on their own.

Before long, the assistance we were called upon to give required more time than we had. In addition, we discovered that what little information has been published on this subject is neither practical nor accurate. These two factors brought us to the realization of the need for this book.

The fear has been expressed that a book which teaches one

how to raise wildlife babies might encourage some people to steal baby animals in order to raise them as pets. In our experience, this fear is groundless. We have had contact with hundreds of people who have adopted and cared for wild babies. Most of them have acquired the babies as the result of legitimate accidents. Their concern is for the welfare of the baby. And they would regard anything less than total freedom, when the time comes, as "cruelty to animals."

The mutual bond of affection which is established between orphan and foster parent remains even after the youngster is given its freedom. The bluejay that has been set free still comes back to visit, landing on your hand for food. The squirrel is equally at home on your shoulder as in the tree. And the raccoon comes around to your house whenever it fishes along the edge of the lake. The experience of raising and freeing an orphan generates an interest in wildlife that seems to last forever. For many young people, the experience has led to a career in wildlife biology, veterinary medicine, or conservation.

WJW

Acknowledgments

I wish to thank:

Mrs. Trudy Farrand, Publishers Services Inc., for her constant encouragement and suggestions.

Dr. Ben Sheffy, Professor of Nutrition and the Assistant Director of the Virus Research Institute at Cornell University, who read an early draft of the manuscript and made excellent suggestions.

Dr. Bill Jackson, a Lakeland, Florida, veterinarian and good friend, who read the text and offered practical comments.

WJW

Contents

Wild Orphan Babies: Mammals and Birds

Introduction

WILDLIFE

Just what is wildlife? In fact, it means different things in different places. In Florida, wildlife includes all wild or non-domesticated birds, mammals, reptiles, and amphibians. What legally constitutes wildlife differs from state to state, as do the laws governing the keeping, holding, and sometimes even helping of wildlife. By law, species such as hawks, owls, mockingbirds, or alligators may not be taken, possessed, harmed, or killed. Thus, these species and many others are given full protection by law.

Wildlife classified as game species is afforded a different kind of protection. Animals such as deer and quail may be hunted, but only at certain times of the year. The law restricts the dates of the hunting season, it limits the time of day, it specifies how these animals may be hunted, and it limits the numbers which may be taken. These wildlife species represent a resource which can be harvested, and this hunting helps keep game animal populations in balance with their available habitat.

There are also species which are classified as unprotected. In Florida, for example, English sparrows, crows, and starlings are not considered valuable, and therefore receive no protection by law. These, along with mice, rats, raccoons, opossums, and armadillos, may be shot, captured, or disposed of in any fashion. While the law does not regard these creatures as valuable, we offer them our help whenever we can, for we enjoy them all.

The law states you may not keep or possess protected wildlife. You must have permission from a game warden or wildlife officer to care for any animal or bird on the protected list. If you acquire an orphan that needs help, the first thing to do is consult a local state wildlife officer or warden. He will tell you if the creature you are trying to help is protected.

Every area of every state has a local game warden or wildlife officer. If you cannot find the officer for your area listed in the telephone directory, call your local police department, sheriff's office, or highway patrol. They will refer you to him.

When you contact the wildlife officer, tell him who you are, the circumstances under which you obtained the orphan or injured creature, what you are planning to do for it, and when you plan to release it. These are sincere, dedicated men who are devoting their lives to helping wildlife. Their advice will therefore be based on what is best for the animal involved. When you have their permission to care for the animal involved, contact your family veterinarian for information on health and professional care.

Additional permission may sometimes be required, as in the case of migratory birds. Birds which migrate across state borders are considered a national asset. They are valuable from an aesthetic point of view, and some, such as ducks, geese, and doves, are also sources of food. The federal government, by agreement with the individual states and the countries of Canada and Mexico, makes the regulations governing these birds. For a list of these birds, see the back of the book.

According to a strict interpretation of the law, you must have a federal permit to keep a bird on this list. However, to confine such a bird temporarily to help with a specific problem, permission from your wildlife officer or warden is usually sufficient.

If, however, you become involved in caring for migratory birds on a year-round basis, you must obtain first a state permit and then an annual federal permit from the Regional Director, Bureau of Sport Fisheries and Wildlife. A list of the Regional Directors appears at the back of the book.

If you find a baby or injured creature on the Rare and Endangered Species list, which includes all the fish, birds, mammals, reptiles, and amphibians in danger of becoming extinct in North America, contact your local wildlife officer. In order to ensure its survival, he will probably want to see that it receives a more professional level of care than you may be able to give. There are presently over one hundred creatures on this list. See the list found at the back of the book.

WARNING TO FOSTER PARENTS

Contact with wild animals can carry an element of risk. Most obvious is the danger of being bitten or scratched.

There is little danger of bite wounds from a tiny orphan if it is given lots of attention and love while growing up. When this baby becomes an adult, however, and the instinct to be with its own kind becomes strong, it can become dangerous. This alone is an excellent reason for raising your orphan to go free.

If you find an injured mature mammal or bird, notify the local wildlife officer of its location and type of injury. Do not try to handle the animal yourself. This is a task only for a professional. Coping with any grown wild animal, such as a raccoon, fox, or otter, is very dangerous. It will bite and can inflict severe injury.

Birds of prey also require caution, for, if frightened, they will defend themselves with their sharp beaks and claws.

A less obvious danger is exposure to disease. To minimize any danger to yourself, follow these basic rules of hygiene:

1. Immediately after you work, play with, or clean up after a wild creature, wash your hands thoroughly with soap and water.

2. Wash any bite wound or scratch thoroughly with soap and water and apply an antiseptic.

3. If an animal dies while you are caring for it, notify your physician or local health department. Based on the information you give, they may or may not suggest further examination.

Few diseases are transmitted directly from birds to man. Based on the experiences of many people in the field, we feel there is little danger.

Of the diseases that can be transmitted from mammals to man, rabies concerns us most. The other communicable diseases represent little practical hazard with the very young animals.

One basic rule is to avoid all wild animals which appear tame. This type of altered or abnormal behavior has always been a sign of rabies in wild animals.

In the last ten years most cases of wildlife rabies have occurred among skunks, raccoons, foxes, and bats. These particular species should, therefore, always be regarded with caution.

In a six-year study conducted by Dr. Paul Schnurrenberger, a public-health veterinarian in Illinois, 911 cases of rabies were diagnosed in wild animals. Fourteen of these animals were being kept as pets at the time. No one died, but several people had to undergo a painful series of injections.

In the Western states a unique hazard exists. Some ground squirrels and prairie dogs carry fleas which are capable of transmitting the organism that causes bubonic plague. For this reason, these ground squirrels and prairie dogs should not be handled. Those which appear tame may be sick, and the fleas leaving these animals can spread plague to people.

While contact with wild animals may carry an element of risk, the care, handling, and raising of wild animals is very satisfying.

Although the information presented in the following pages can also be used to raise an orphan puppy or kitten, I have not included these and other common pets because information on caring for them is available from your local veterinarian. Nor have I included frogs, toads, snakes, and other amphibians and reptiles. From the time of hatching they have the ability to care for themselves and do not require assistance.

Mammals

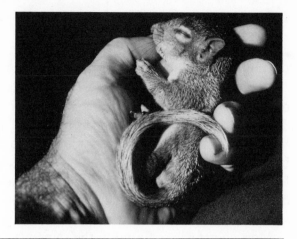

1

Basic Care of Orphan Mammals

WHAT IS AN ORPHAN?

There are two types of orphans: animals which have lost their mothers and are too young to survive on their own; and animals which, though physically old enough to care for themselves, cannot do so because they have been weakened or injured.

It is commonly believed that once a human being has touched a wild baby, its mother will abandon it. In most cases, this is not true. Babies should not be handled, but for a different reason: they may flee from you and get lost or hurt trying to escape.

A fully furred orphan that can walk rather than crawl and whose eyes are open and bright is usually old enough to care for itself, even though it may be tiny. Be kind. Leave this baby in the wild where it belongs. However, a cold, wet baby whose eyes are not yet open needs help. A baby in danger because of the family cat or other predator should also be rescued.

Babies are orphaned in different ways. Most often they are orphaned when their mother is injured or killed in an accident. Sometimes a raccoon mother is killed and the babies she has left high in a tree will grow hungry and begin to cry. Such babies should be rescued. Or an injured raccoon baby may be found on the ground, having fallen or crawled from its tree den. If there is no way to put it back in the den, and the mother is nowhere around, the baby will have to be adopted.

Most squirrels are found in the same way. "Drays," or nests built of twigs and leaves high in a tree, sometimes come apart in a storm, and tiny baby squirrels are found cold and wet under the tree.

Baby rabbits are also frequently found after a storm. The mother rabbit builds her nest in a shallow depression in the grass. When a heavy rain floods the nest, the babies will often crawl to higher ground.

In spring and summer an opossum that has been killed in an accident should be checked to see if she has babies with her. If very tiny, they would be found in the pouch on the mother's abdomen, and if large enough to have their eyes open and to have hair, they would more likely be found clinging to the fur on her back.

APPROACHING THE BABY

A very small baby that has no hair or whose eyes are not yet open may be picked up in your bare hands. Gently slide your fingers under the baby, scoop it up, and cradle it in your palms. Most babies, particularly very small ones, will enjoy the warmth of your hands. Adjust your fingers to fit snugly around the baby, so it can absorb the maximum warmth from your fingers, but not so snugly that it can't shift its posi-

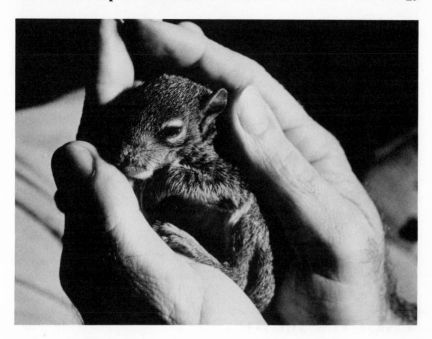

Cupped hands serve as warm substitute nest for gray squirrel.

tion. The tiny, hairless baby will become quiet almost at once and will soon drop off to sleep.

The larger baby should be approached more cautiously. Do not sneak up on it silently, as a predator might. Talk to the baby in a low, soothing voice, and it will have the confidence to let you come close. The baby will be less frightened if you stoop, or in some way come lower to its level, rather than if you tower over it like a giant. When you are close enough, offer your hand for the baby to smell. Do not extend a finger, in case it should attempt to bite. If it doesn't try to bite and seems quite satisfied with the first step you have taken in getting acquainted, slowly change the position of your hand so you can stroke its back, petting it as you would a kitten, only more slowly and more gently.

Be wary until you see how your offer of friendship is received. If the baby tries to bite you when you touch it, start over again. First let it smell your hand, then try to stroke it gently. If it accepts being stroked, then you can try to pick it up.

It is wise to wear gloves or to protect yourself in some other way. If you don't have gloves with you, use your shirt or jacket instead. Open it and place one hand under it. Use the other hand, covered with part of the shirt, to "herd" or push the baby to your outstretched, waiting hand. Move your hands together gently under the baby until one hand is on either side of it, forming a nest in which to carry it. Place a fold of the shirt or jacket over the baby to prevent it from jumping out and injuring itself. As the baby absorbs the warmth of your hands, you have taken the first step in the basic care that will keep it alive.

A NEST FOR THE BABY

To provide warmth and security, the first requirements of care for all very young animals, transfer the baby from your hands to a nest box as soon as possible. Any box the size of a shoe box, lined with cotton, flannel, or a piece of an old sweater, will make a fine nest. The material must be soft and comfortable in order to simulate the mother's nest. The sides of the nest should be high enough so the baby won't accidentally fall out. The baby must have room enough to move around so it can get into a comfortable position. Tiny babies can only turn around by crawling forward.

KEEPING THE BABY WARM

Place the nest box in an area free from drafts. An ordinary 60-watt light bulb will provide adequate heat and warmth for the newborn or very young baby. Hang the light bulb near the

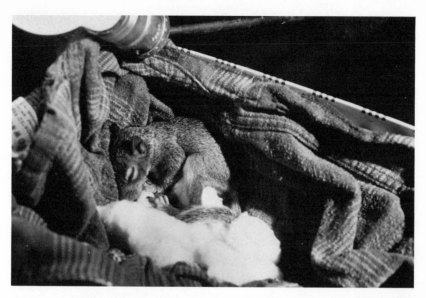

A nest made from an old shoebox, a flannel shirt, and a light bulb is used for young, tiny mammal babies.

nest using an extension cord, like a mechanic's trouble light, or use a flexible gooseneck study lamp. Position the light over one end of the nest, so the temperature will vary from one end to the other. This will enable the baby to move closer to the light when it is cold and farther away when it feels too warm. Place an inexpensive outdoor thermometer in or beside the nest.

By knowing a little about the species of animal you have adopted, you can make a rough estimate of its age. Many mammals, such as squirrels, are born without hair, while some, such as cats, are born already covered with soft, fine hair. All are born with the eyes sealed closed. The hairless babies begin growing hair at once. Within fourteen to twenty-four days after birth, the hairless babies have hair and in almost all mammal babies the eyes have opened.

For the very young hairless baby, adjust the light or the nest until you have a temperature of 95° F.

If the baby has some hair but the eyes are still closed, maintain a temperature of 90° F. until the eyes open. Once the eyes open, drop the temperature of the nest 5° F. each week.

You should have no problem keeping a young baby in the nest. They seem to appreciate the warmth and the security that a comfortable nest affords. A light burning continuously doesn't bother them. They know no darkness, or night as such, and readily accept the light as part of their world.

How long should bulb heat be provided? When you see that the baby no longer sleeps near the bulb or snuggles up close to it after play, you can remove it. The baby no longer needs warmth from this source.

Caution: The temperature-control mechanism of a baby's body functions poorly. It is easy to kill a baby with too much heat. This has happened when heating pads were used to provide heat and the baby couldn't escape from the excessive warmth. Older babies can compensate for a while by panting, but the very young aren't able to eliminate excessive body heat this way. If you must use a heating pad temporarily, leave room for the baby to crawl off it. Use your thermometer to watch the temperature closely.

The temperature-regulating mechanism of the baby's body begins to function more efficiently about the time the eyes begin to open. When this happens, accurate temperature monitoring of the nest is less critical, but still important if the baby is to be kept comfortable.

Warming a Chilled Baby

Never warm a chilled or cold baby too rapidly. A heat lamp, heating pad, or even the light bulb will not warm the baby uniformly. The body surface will warm at once, but the internal structures will remain cool longer. The warm outer tissues demand more nutrients and oxygen. But the baby's heart, which is beating weakly and slowly because of its low tem-

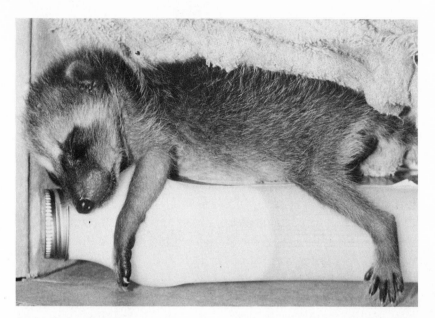

A plastic bottle filled with warm water temporarily keeps a baby raccoon warm.

perature (hypothermia), is unable to supply these. By the time the internal structures are warm and the heart stronger, the outer warm tissues are badly damaged. The accumulation of waste products and the poisons of tissue breakdown entering the system of the weakened baby are enough to cause its death.

The chilled baby should therefore be warmed very gradually with your body heat. Cradle the baby in your hands until it feels warm to your touch. This may take two to three hours, or longer. Of if it is tiny, put the baby in a shirt pocket under your sweater, or just hold it in your lap while you read a book or watch television. When it becomes active and no longer feels cold, place it in its shoe-box nest. We often place a plastic bottle filled with warm water in the nest box. The baby will snuggle up to the warm bottle, drawing both heat and comfort from its presence.

BOWEL AND URINE CONTROL

The nest box rarely has to be cleaned, because you control the elimination of the tiny baby. When it is a little older, it will leave the nest to eliminate.

Controlling bowel and urine eliminations in the very young is not a matter of choice. It is a necessity. The very young baby, hairless and with its eyes closed, will not normally defecate or urinate on its own. It is stimulated to do so by its mother by licking. Since you have taken over the duties of the mother you must stimulate urination. Take a small piece of cotton about the size of a fifty-cent piece. Moisten it with comfortably warm water and squeeze out the excess. Cradle the baby in one hand as it lies on its back, and gently stroke the genital organs with the warm moist cotton. After three to ten quick, gentle strokes, the baby will begin to urinate. Tiny drops of liquid will appear on the genital organs after each stroke. Continue stroking until the flow ceases. The mother stimulates bowel movements, or defecation, in the same fashion, and so must you. Most babies will urinate and defecate each time they are fed. Take care of this chore before each feeding so you aren't "messed upon" during the feeding. Having these two functions under your control helps keep the baby and its nest clean and neat.

When a baby reaches two to four weeks of age, it no longer needs your stimulation to eliminate. However, continue to make it eliminate before you feed or handle it for as long as you can. As it gets older, the baby acquires voluntary control over elimination, and it will take over the function itself.

If you acquire the baby after its eyes are open, you ordinarily cannot stimulate bowel or urine elimination since the older baby already has control over the act. You can try, however. If you are successful, keep control of this function as long as you can. If unsuccessful, you will have a messier baby, but not necessarily a messier nest. If the baby can leave the nest to eliminate, it will usually do so. If it can eliminate but can't get out, it will probably eliminate when you take it from its nest to feed it. After the first couple of "accidents," you will form the habit of placing a tissue or paper towel under the "accident" end during feeding and handling. Once the baby has eliminated, you will be able to play with it safely for several hours.

HOUSES AND CAGES

When the baby begins to crawl out of the nest regularly, it is time for more permanent housing. Needed now are two things: a house and a cage.

The Nest-Box House

This simple wooden structure is intended as a semipermanent home. The orphan will use it while it is growing into a mature animal and even after it has its freedom, so the nest box must be large enough to accommodate an adult animal. Only when the orphan goes back to the wild permanently will it give up this home.

Construct it from any durable wood scraps that can withstand rain and weather when it is moved outdoors. It is better if it is not painted. Many paints contain materials which are toxic.

A mouse or flying squirrel will need a house with dimensions of $4'' \times 4'' \times 6''$ with an entrance hole 1 inch in diameter. A house for a medium-sized animal, such as a gray squirrel, should have inside dimensions of $8'' \times 8'' \times 8''$ with a 2-inch entrance hole. A large orphan, such as a fox, skunk, or raccoon, needs a house with inside dimensions of $12'' \times 12'' \times 18''$ with an entrance hole 6 inches in diameter.

The house should have a hinged or removable top. This will

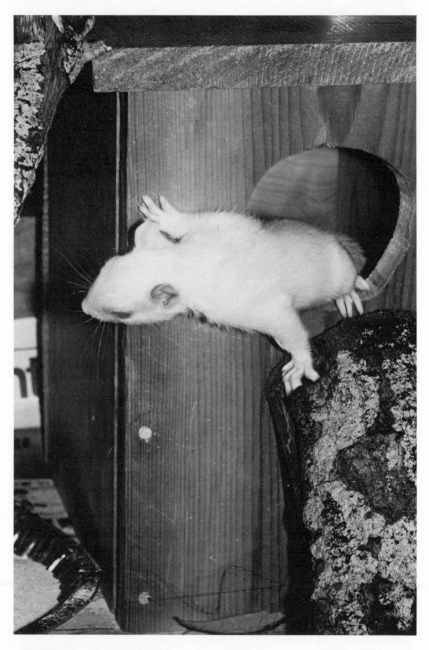

An albino gray squirrel in its nest-box-house.

make it easy to remove the orphan and also to clean the nest.

Transfer the bedding from the original nest to the new nest-box house. Add to this enough new bedding to line the house adequately. The familiar bedding, even in new surroundings, will make the change easier for the baby. The nest-box house is placed inside the cage.

The Cage

The cage is made from galvanized wire mesh called hardware cloth. Any hardware store sells it. Get a 30-inch-wide piece about 12 feet long and a spool of fine wire. Cut the hardware cloth with a tin snips and bend it with your hands to form the cage sides. Use the fine wire to lace the sides and top together. The door can be fabricated of hardware cloth and wired in place as part of one side of the cage.

A cage can never be too large. The minimum size for a mouse or flying squirrel is $18'' \times 24'' \times 24''$, and for a gray squirrel, $30'' \times 36'' \times 36''$. A fox, skunk, or raccoon requires a

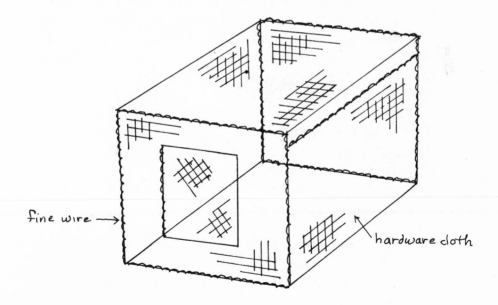

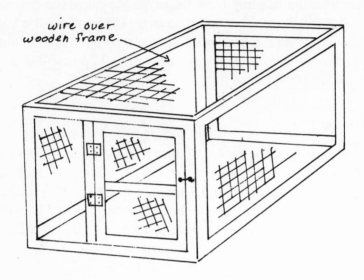

really large house, 48″ × 48″ × 48″. A cage as large as that is best made by tacking hardware cloth over a wooden frame.

The cage must be large enough for the baby to have room to run, climb, romp, and play. Wire a series of limbs, an inch or so in diameter, around the inside of the cage and to each other in order to create a jungle gym for the baby to climb about on. This will ensure a happier and healthier baby with good, sturdy muscles.

When you place the nest home in the cage, you can discontinue using the light bulb for warmth, if you haven't done so before. If there is any doubt about whether to continue it now, place the bulb either in the cage or against the wire outside of it, so warmth is available if the orphan wants it. When the baby no longer seeks the warmth of the bulb and ignores it, remove it.

Line the bottom of the cage with newspapers. At this age the orphan will always leave the nest box to urinate and to eliminate bowel material in the bottom of the cage. Change the paper as needed, which is usually every other day. With smaller babies, such as flying squirrels and baby rabbits, there isn't much "mess" to be cleaned up. Use your own judgment to determine when the cage needs cleaning. It is better to clean it too often than not often enough. Bowel material accidentally swallowed by the baby as it cleans and grooms itself can cause intestinal infection, diarrhea, and even death. Cleanliness is one of the most important factors in raising a healthy, happy baby.

Once the baby becomes active enough to play and romp about in the new cage, give it the freedom of a screened porch and part of the house. At our house, cages are used primarily for sleeping and feeding. We let the babies out in the morning and give them the run of the back screened porch and part of the house during the day. Cages never represent confinement to the babies, but rather a place of rest and security. With the freedom to come and go, they don't resent being placed in them and accept the cage as home.

WATER

Once the nest home is placed in a cage and the baby is actively moving about, supply a source of water. For small creatures such as squirrels, wire a water bottle with a sipper tube (this can be obtained at any pet store) to the side of the cage. For larger animals, place a dish of water in a corner of the cage. Keep the water dish clean and be sure to supply fresh water daily.

Tiny babies in a nest are not given water since, as you shall see, they receive all the fluid they need in their formula.

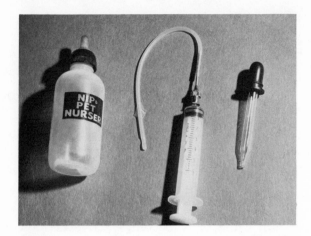

2

Feeding Orphan Mammals

WHEN TO START FEEDING

Now that the baby is comfortable, warm, and no longer frightened, it will be hungry. It is now time to consider feeding.

Do not try to feed the orphan until its body temperature has been brought back to normal. A chilled baby cannot digest food. The chilled baby is cold to the touch and is inactive. The baby with a normal body temperature will move about and feel warm to the touch. You may see it start nuzzling the nest material or begin to crawl and search about the nest. This is the time to start feeding.

THE FORMULA

All young babies are fed a formula as a substitute for its mother's milk. Essentially, the formula consists of homogenized milk and egg yolk.

Prepare 6 to 8 ounces of formula at a time. Mix the formula in a clean bowl with a fork, rotary beater, or in a blender. Transfer it to a clean jar, cover and refrigerate. Remove only enough for one feeding at a time. Pour the formula into a clean glass or measuring cup, and warm it by placing the glass in a bowl of warm water.

Test the temperature by dropping a few drops on your wrist. If it feels barely warm, it is the correct temperature. If it feels warm or hot, it is too hot and should not be used until it cools down.

We use varying combinations of homogenized milk and egg yolk to prepare a formula similar to the mother's milk. Egg yolk is an excellent source of protein. It is easily digested and is rich in vitamins A and D and fatty acids. It adds fat and protein to those present in the milk, making a suitable formula for most mammal babies.* See the back of the book for the composition of milk.

---

* The amounts of food required by an orphan can be figured in calories, which are units of energy. A newborn kitten (this would be close enough for squirrels, raccoons, opossums, and even for fox puppies) requires 250 calories per kilogram of body weight per day. Or, in figures we are more used to considering, this would be 100 calories per pound per day to meet its energy requirements. The basic formula as we mix it contains approximately 28 to 30 calories per ounce. We consider an egg yolk to contain 60 calories and milk, 20.6 calories per ounce. This means a kitten weighing 1 pound (16 ounces) would need about 4 ounces of formula daily.

The requirements of a squirrel or mouse would be higher because of the higher rate of body metabolism. If for the sake of a starting point we say the requirements for the squirrel would be 150 calories per pound or 10 calories per ounce, a 3-ounce squirrel would require 30 calories daily. This is about 1 ounce or 30 cc. of the *concentrated* formula, since each ounce of the more concentrated formula contains 30 to 35 calories. Each dropper delivers ½ cc. per dose which would mean sixty droppers daily or over ten droppers in each of six feedings. We have rarely seen a squirrel that size take that much. This points up the weakness of attempting to make hard and fast feeding rules, and indicates the need for you to use common sense and judgment in your feeding programs.

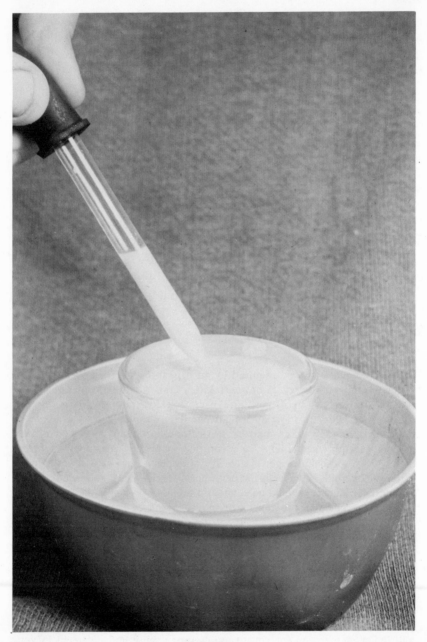

Warming formula in a bowl of warm water.

Formula for Babies Which Will Be Small As Adults, Such As Mice, Flying Squirrels, Gray Squirrels, and Kittens

These babies require a concentrated formula. Usually, the smaller the animal, the higher its rate of metabolism, and the more calories (energy) it requires. Since it both eats less and has a greater need for energy, formula must be rich for them. Mix one large egg yolk in sufficient milk to make 4 to 6 ounces of formula, or one half to three fourths of a cup.

FORMULA FOR BABY RABBITS.   These babies may be fed exactly as above with the exception that antibiotics may be added to their formula once their eyes are open. For more information on this subject, see the section on antibiotics in the next chapter.

Caution: No other baby mammals should routinely receive antibiotics.

Formula for Babies Which Will Grow into Large Adults, Such As Opossums, Raccoons, and Foxes

Use one large egg yolk or two small egg yolks and add enough homogenized milk to make 8 ounces or one cup of formula. This is the basic formula.

Formula for Larger Mammals, Such As Baby Goats and Deer

Use one egg yolk in sufficient milk to make 8 ounces. When these animals are two weeks of age, make the formula one egg yolk to 12 ounces of milk, and when they are four weeks old, increase it to one egg yolk in 16 ounces (1 pint) of milk. Deer and goats do well on this formula. When they begin to take a pint per feeding, substitute powdered non-fat skim milk for homogenized milk. Use more milk than the directions on the package call for. If package directions say add one and one third cups of powdered milk to enough water to make a quart, use two cups of milk instead. Care of deer, wild goats, wild sheep, or antelope would be very temporary, since all state game commissions have facilities for professional care and insist that these species be turned over to them.

Sweetener

While the simple formula of milk and egg yolk is adequate for all common mammals, a sweetener may sometimes be added for better results.

For any baby that doesn't take to the formula, add a little honey. One level teaspoon to the formula combination does not change the caloric content significantly but does make it a little sweeter. Sometimes a stubborn formula-taker becomes an enthusiastic eater when fed the sweeter formula. Once you start adding honey to the formula, you will have to continue using it, for the baby will not accept the less tasty formula from then on. It is amusing to watch a baby that has had honey being offered the formula without this ingredient. It will begin to suck the formula greedily but will spit it out after the first taste. Its whole attitude is one of disgust, and it resists any further offers of the unsweetened formula.

WAYS OF FEEDING FORMULA

Two different feeding techniques are commonly used, depending upon the age and size of the baby. One is by bottle, the other by medicine dropper.

Dropper Feeding

The most effective way to feed the very young and the very small orphan is with a medicine dropper. A tiny mouse baby, ½ inch long, or a large almost weaned rabbit can be fed

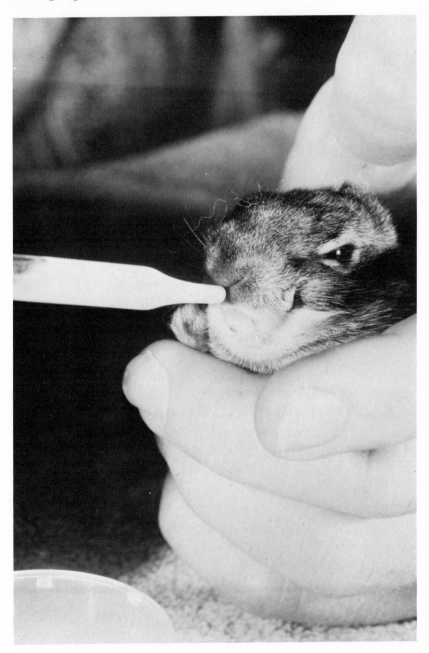

Dropper feeding of a baby rabbit.

equally effectively with a dropper. Some babies do not have the strength to suck on a nipple and bottle. Many babies won't even try. With the dropper, you can force small amounts of the formula into the mouth. Also, with dropper feeding, you can more easily tell if the baby is getting food.

When you are ready to feed the baby, fill your dropper with formula. Hold the baby in the palm of your hand with the head end slightly higher than the rear quarters. The head should be almost horizontal. Do not tilt it up too high. This will stretch the muscles of the throat, and the baby will be unable to swallow.

With the baby in the proper position in one hand and the dropper in the other hand, gently force the dropper just inside the lips. Do not place it deep within the mouth. Pressing the bulb of the dropper gently, release a tiny amount of liquid into the baby's mouth. In all but the very weakest baby this will stimulate a licking motion. A stronger baby will actually grasp the end of the dropper with its lips and start sucking. If it licks and swallows, or begins to suck on the dropper, you can give a silent cheer; the challenge of raising an orphan is half won.

As the baby licks or sucks, you can help it by pressing *very slowly* on the rubber bulb and gradually expelling the contents of the dropper as the baby swallows. If bubbles appear at the baby's nose, or if it opens its mouth very wide (a gagging motion), you are expelling the formula too rapidly. The baby cannot handle the amount you have given it. Remove the dropper and tilt the head down, so the formula can drain out of the mouth, throat, and nose. Wipe the excess formula from the face with a tissue. Give the baby a few moments to recover, then once again start feeding, only this time more slowly.

When the baby has finished eating and the dropper is emptied, use a tissue to wipe the excess formula from the baby's lips and chin. Keeping the baby clean as you feed it keeps the hair around its head and neck from becoming encrusted with dried formula, which will become sour-smelling.

Refill the dropper and repeat the procedure as long as the baby will accept the formula. As the baby becomes stronger and you become more proficient, you will quickly adapt your ability to give formula to its ability to take it. Each baby varies in the way in which it accepts the feeding procedure, which means you have to learn the best and most effective way for your individual orphan baby.

Some babies, particularly those whose eyes are already open, will often take the formula best if fed drop by drop in the following way: hang one drop of formula at a time on the tip of the dropper and let the baby lick it off; replace it with another drop each time the baby licks it off. This method works particularly well for baby rabbits.

How much food the baby is consuming tells a lot about the condition of your orphan. If at each feeding it takes a little more than the time before, you are making progress.

Once the baby accepts the formula and recognizes it as food, it will usually accept each succeeding dropperful more readily. When it sucks greedily on the end of the dropper, you can change to a bottle.

How much to feed. The amount to feed depends upon the size and condition of the baby. A baby squirrel with no hair, 1½ inches long, may take only two to ten drops at a feeding. An older squirrel, 3 or 4 inches long, which has hair but whose eyes are closed, will more likely take two to six dropperfuls. A squirrel 4 inches long with its eyes open would take from four to ten dropperfuls at each feeding.

The amount and frequency of feeding will vary but are related. A squirrel 3 inches long, furred, but with its eyes closed, which is strong when you find it, will probably take three to six dropperfuls, sucking vigorously and hungrily. But the same squirrel which was badly chilled and is now warmed but still weak will probably take only one half a dropperful of

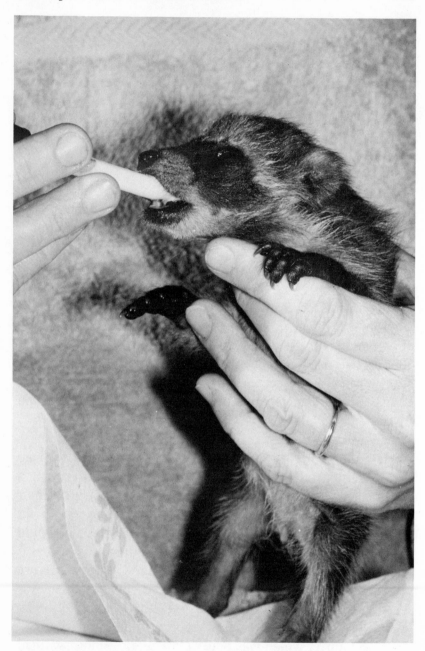

Baby raccoon eats greedily.

formula. The strong squirrel may be satisfied if fed every two or three hours. The weak squirrel should be fed every thirty minutes, in the hope that it will eat a little more each time. When it gets stronger and eats normally, it will eat enough at one time to satisfy its hunger for several hours.

This variation in amounts is true regardless of species. A weak, tiny mouse or flying squirrel will take only one or two drops. A healthy orphan, the same size, might take as much as a quarter dropperful. When a wild baby has had enough, you just can't get it to take any more. After the first few days you will know how often the baby will accept food.

With a little experience, you will often be able to tell whether the baby is ready to eat by watching it for a few moments. The full, contented baby sleeps rather quietly. You may see a little involuntary twitching, which is perfectly normal. The hungry baby is restless. It will raise its head and creep about the nest area every few seconds. The hungry, older baby with its eyes open will be standing in the nest or peering over the edge looking for food. These are your signals that it is time for the next feeding.

Basically, let your orphan tell you how much it wants to eat and when. If it eats less than you expect, you can anticipate that it will be hungry again soon. Most babies want to eat about four times daily and will stop eating when they have had enough.

Therefore, feed only as much as the baby wants. Offer food frequently until you have learned something of your orphan's eating habits and its eating pattern is established.

Bottle Feeding

Larger babies, such as deer and goats, are taught from the start to eat from an infant nursing bottle. Smaller babies are changed over to bottle feeding when they are consuming an ounce or more of formula at each feeding. Because of the stiff

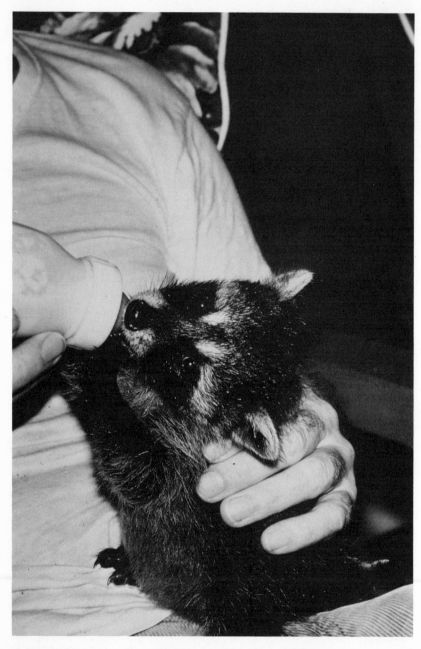

An older baby raccoon is fed with a baby bottle.

nipple, doll bottles are usually not satisfactory for small animals. A baby-animal bottle (Nip-Pet Nurser), which may be obtained from a veterinarian or pet store, works well for small animals. Use a small infant nursing bottle with a "preemie" nipple after the orphan weighs a pound or more. These are purchased at a drugstore.

Since the egg yolk formula is thicker than most prepared milk formulas, the openings in the end of any new nipple must be enlarged for nursing an orphan baby. Pass a heated needle through the existing hole, or enlarge the hole to small slits with a sharp knife. If the nipple has a tendency to plug up, filter the formula through several layers of gauze. This will remove any lumps of yolk material that might stop up the nipple.

How MUCH TO FEED.   Most babies will be bottle-fed three to four times daily. Fill the bottle with the amount of formula the baby will consume at one feeding. You will soon learn how much formula it takes to satisfy your baby at each feeding.

Start with 4 to 6 ounces of formula two to three times daily for a young tiny fawn, and increase the amount as it grows.

After bottle feeding, the baby should be "burped." Hold it in an almost upright position in your hand. Pat its back gently to "coax" out any swallowed air. A larger baby can be placed on your shoulder as a human infant would be and patted in the same way. With hoofed animals, such as deer and goats, this is not necessary.

Weaning the Baby

Most babies wean themselves. They give up the dropper or bottle of formula when they begin eating other foods well. However, some just don't like to give it up. They seem not only to enjoy the formula as food, but also the companionship and attention they receive at feeding time. Even some adult animals enjoy a bottle of formula. We don't force weaning but feed the formula as long as the orphan desires it.

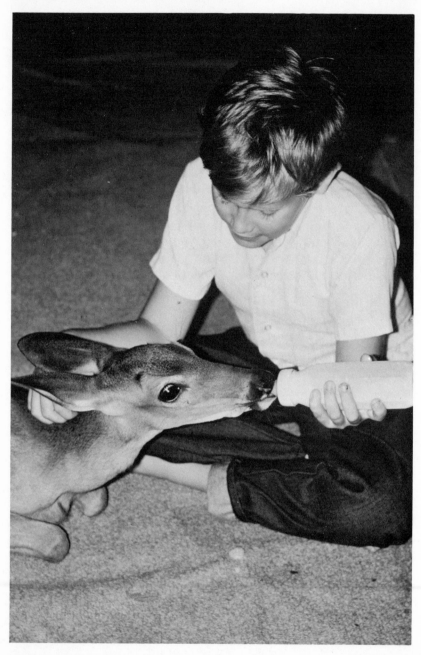

Deer being fed formula from bottle.

Stomach-Tube Feeding

This is for the problem baby. The weak baby that refuses
to eat from the dropper, or does not have the strength to suck
or the will to swallow, must be fed by stomach tube. Chances
are you will not have to do this. Such a baby is not often
found. But if you should find and adopt one, it is well to be
prepared. This procedure is safe, easy, and effective. You
can easily accomplish it on your own. If you have any ques-
tions, though, consult your veterinarian.

EQUIPMENT.   The necessary equipment will have to be obtained from your veterinarian. You will need a small plastic
syringe and a piece of plastic tubing. For most babies, such as
squirrels, raccoons, and foxes, tubing ⅛ inch in diameter and
6 or 8 inches long will work best. Your veterinarian will help
you select the size syringe and tubing most appropriate for
your baby and demonstrate how to use them. Attach the
syringe to the tubing. Fill the syringe with formula.

HOW FAR TO BABY'S STOMACH?   Before you can place the
contents of the syringe directly into the stomach, which sounds
more difficult than it is, first measure the distance from baby's
mouth to the stomach. Hold the tube alongside the baby,
putting the tip of the tube just past the baby's last rib. With
a Magic Marker or pen, mark the tube at the nose point. This
is the distance to the baby's stomach. When you insert the
tube and the mark reaches the baby's lips, you will know the
end is in the stomach.

THE FEEDING PROCESS.   When you are ready to feed, place
the baby on its stomach on a table or counter. Place your left
hand around its body, your thumb near the mouth and forefinger on the other side of the head. Gently insert the tips of
your thumb and forefinger into the baby's mouth, forcing it
slightly open. Moisten the tube with a little formula for
lubrication, and insert the tube over the tongue, aiming for the
deepest part of the throat. Gently slide the tube down into the

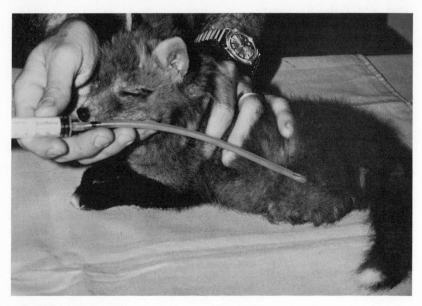

Baby fox being measured for stomach-tube feeding.

stomach. When the "nosemark" is even with the lips, you are there.

All your movements should be gentle. If the tube appears to stop, or doesn't go in readily, withdraw it slightly and then continue. The trachea or windpipe presents no problem. Do not try to avoid it. The tube will go down the right place. If the tube doesn't go to the "nosemark," or if for one reason or another you aren't sure, remove the tube, moisten it with formula again, and start over.

HOW MUCH TO FEED.   Once the tube is in place, press the syringe very gently and slowly release a small amount of formula into the baby's stomach. If this goes well, press again and give about one fourth the total amount. Pause for five or six seconds to be sure the baby is handling it, then give one half of the remainder. Pause again, and give the balance. When the formula is gone, remove the tube.

Stomach-tube feeding four times a day is sufficient, since more is given at each feeding than with the medicine dropper.

Still, watch for "hungry" signals and feed as your orphan needs it. Since the medicine-dropper method is safer, and since the baby helps and participates in it rather than just being a passive "blob" that you are manipulating, switch to the dropper as soon as possible.

GAGGING.   The gagging reflex is not well developed in very young babies. Therefore, it will not interfere with the feeding process. Nor will the baby attempt to get rid of the tube. Since the tube may interfere slightly with breathing, however, don't leave it in any longer than necessary. The gagging reflex develops after the baby's eyes open, and at this age tube feeding is not necessary, except in sick or very weak babies.

If you squirt the formula into the stomach too rapidly, the baby will not be able to handle it, and vomiting will occur. This rarely happens, but if it does, withdraw the tube immediately, hold the baby in a head-down position, and gently pat it over the back and chest area, just as a mother would a human infant. This helps clear the chest of any liquid which might have been sucked into the trachea.

VETERINARY ASSISTANCE.   If your veterinarian demonstrates stomach-tube feeding for you, he may use a clear liquid that contains a little sugar and essential salts. This sugar solution is used for the first one or two feedings when the baby is dehydrated (a lack of water in the tissues and circulatory system). The solution is also used when the baby is too weak to accept regular formula. Ordinarily you should not have to use it. Tell your veterinarian that you intend to use the basic egg yolk and milk formula. If he suggests changing it for a few days to combat a specific problem, follow his advice.

If there is no veterinarian in your community, study the illustrations of the feeding utensils and make your own adaptations as best you can. You may find it easier than you expect, and you may save a baby that would otherwise have been lost. Veterinary medicine, and all medicine, has one basic rule: *DO NO HARM.* If it appears that what you are attempting to do might do damage to the baby—don't do it.

Washing Up

Cleanliness is essential for a healthy baby.

Any bacteria present in the warmed formula will grow rapidly and could make the orphan baby sick. Therefore, discard all uneaten formula.

After feeding, clean all utensils thoroughly. Wash them first in cold water, to loosen milk particles, then in very hot water. Place them on a clean paper napkin or paper towel and allow them to air-dry. They will then be clean and ready for the next use.

Detergents should not be necessary. If, however, you did not have an opportunity to clean your utensils after feeding and the milk has dried and hardened, wash them in detergent. Be sure to rinse them thoroughly, for any detergent left on the utensil will make the baby sick. They may be sanitized and disinfected by adding a small amount of Clorox to the final rinse water.

Intestinal upsets caused by detergents or by infection from dirty utensils probably cause more deaths when raising orphan babies than any other factor. The baby's intestinal tract is very sensitive, and in the baby under ten days of age the intestines allow bacteria and poisons to enter its system.

FOODS FOR THE OLDER BABY

As your orphan baby gets older, it will leave the nest to play and explore. This is the time to add other foods to its diet.

Baby cereal, such as Gerber's oatmeal or Hi-Protein cereal, and baby food may be added to its formula to make it more nutritious and satisfying. Just remember that the openings in the nipple must be made even larger to accommodate this thicker formula.

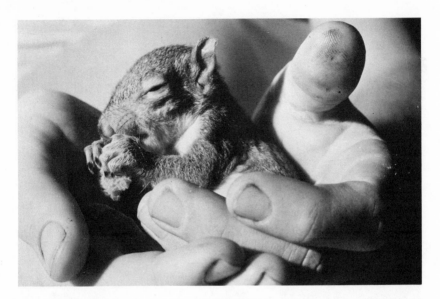

Gray squirrel eats first solid food, dry breakfast cereal.

Flying Squirrels, Squirrels, and Mice

Offer these babies dry breakfast cereals and nuts as their first new foods. Most babies will accept unsweetened oat and wheat cereals. The baby squirrel will usually grasp a piece of cereal in both hands and bite little pieces out of it. Of all the nuts, shelled pecans are the favorite. As soon as the baby is eating nuts well, discontinue the cereal. Continue to feed the formula along with the nuts. Add fruits and other new foods daily. Grapes, orange sections, pieces of apple, lettuce leaves, bits of brown bread, carrots, and any other fruits should be offered if they are available.

If acorns and other seeds that squirrels would normally eat in the wild are available, offer these as well. The sooner these wild creatures begin eating the food they will eat when they are free, the easier will be their transition back to the wild.

Do not try to supply all the foods that an animal would find in the wild. Some animals eat foods such as grasshoppers and

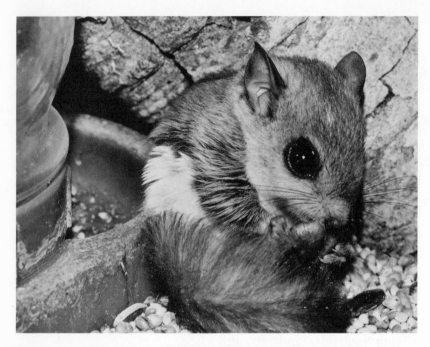

A variety of foods for baby flying squirrel.

other large bugs which are too difficult to obtain. Others are predators who eat smaller creatures such as mice, rats, and rabbits. We feel it is not right for us to kill one animal to sustain another.

Baby Rabbits

Start with dry breakfast food and any green leafy vegetables. Rabbits normally start eating green plant foods at a very early age. When the babies are old enough to start hopping around the cage, offer bits of lettuce, celery leaves, cabbage, apples, and any green plants they will find outdoors.

There are so many foods available to rabbits when they are given their freedom that their dietary transition is not at all difficult. As they eat more of the items you offer, they will take less and less of the formula. When they don't want the formula any more and you have to coax them to take it, it is time to give them their freedom.

Fox Puppies, Skunks, Opossums, Raccoons, and Bobcats

When they are old enough to become playful, usually about four or five weeks of age, offer a little bowl of a complete canned dog food mixed with an equal amount of formula.

CANNED DOG FOOD. A complete canned dog food is a high-quality, balanced food that has met the nutritional requirements of the National Research Council, Washington, D.C. This would be indicated on the label. The label should further state that the contents constitute a complete and balanced diet for a dog. This food, a mixture of meat and cereal grains, should have a meaty consistency and odor. One that is oily, greasy, or has a musty, unpleasant odor should not be used. All-meat dog foods should not be used, because they often cause diarrhea in the young orphan.

Mix the dog food with enough formula to make it the consistency of thick soup or oatmeal, and offer it on your finger. If the baby licks your finger, offer it the entire bowl. As the baby begins to eat more of the dog food-formula combination, it will become less interested in eating formula from the bottle or dropper. Once it is eating well, gradually discontinue feeding the formula and offer only the dog food-formula mixture four to six times daily. Discard what the baby hasn't eaten after five or ten minutes, as a great deal of bacterial growth can take place within a few hours in moist food standing at room temperature. Over the next ten days gradually reduce the amount of formula in the mixture until you are feeding just canned dog food.

DRY FOOD. When the baby is eating canned food well, introduce it to dry cat or dog food. As long as the label states that the dry food is a complete, balanced food, either cat or

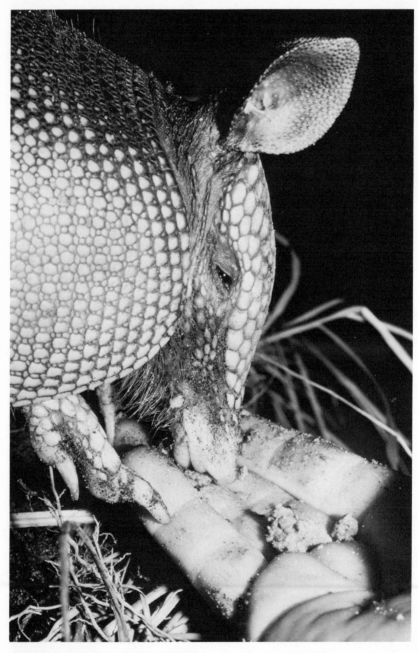

Armadillo eating canned dog food.

dog food is satisfactory. Skunks, opossums, armadillos, and cats are usually fed dry cat food. The other species are given dry dog food. Leave a bowl of dry food in the cage at all times for the orphan to snack on. When it begins eating it well, gradually reduce the amount and frequency of the canned dog food feedings.

It is important to change an orphan from the canned to the dry food. Since dry food does not spoil readily, it is easier to keep this food available when the baby is free.

While the dry food will be its basic diet, continue to offer the orphan a variety of foods. Individual babies often show decided food preferences, and it is most interesting to see what a new orphan will like and accept.

Any creature normally has a varied diet in the wild. It is abnormal for an orphan to eat one particular food to the exclusion of all others. If it does, in time it will develop a deficiency. The easiest way to handle this problem is to withdraw the preferred food and offer alternative foods until the baby is eating these other foods well. You may then return the withdrawn food to the diet, but only in small amounts.

DIET SUPPLEMENTS

Dietary supplements are usually added to a diet to make up for a deficiency. The most common dietary supplements are vitamin-mineral preparations. It is not necessary to add a vitamin supplement to the basic milk and egg yolk formula, as this food contains high-quality protein and adequate vitamins and minerals. Nor is it necessary to add supplements to a good canned dog food or dry chow. They have already been supplied with vitamins and minerals.

Cod-liver oil is a widely recommended dietary supplement in animal and bird publications. However, to add it to the diet is to risk permanent damage to your orphan. Cod-liver oil primarily supplies vitamins A and D and affects calcium utilization. In high dosages these vitamins are toxic.

Since vitamin D is the more toxic, it concerns us most. In large amounts, vitamin D increases the level of calcium in the blood. However, unless additional calcium and phosphorus are provided in proper balance in the diet, the vitamin D maintains this higher blood level by drawing calcium from the animal's bones. Prolonged use of cod-liver oil leads to what is called "demineralization" of the skeleton, which simply means the bones lose their density and strength as they lose their calcium. Multiple fractures, bending, and twisting of the bones become commonplace. High calcium levels in the blood also cause damage to blood vessels and kidneys.

The percentage of carbohydrates, fats, and proteins required in the diets of most wild animals is known, but specific information on essential amino acids and vitamin and mineral requirements has not been established. We do know, however, that all these creatures require vitamins and minerals, just as humans do. Our basic formula provides them in adequate amounts.

A neat, healthy appearance in an active orphan is the best evidence that it is being adequately supplied with the vitamins and minerals it requires. As long as an orphan is eating well and eating a variety of foods, extra vitamins and minerals are not necessary.

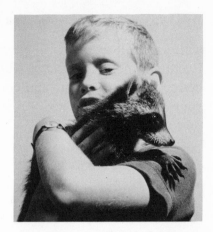

3

Petting, Handling, and Freedom

PETTING AND HANDLING

Contrary to what you might expect, an orphan should receive a great deal of petting, handling, and attention. After feeding, hold the baby for a little while in your cupped hands. It will burrow around for a few moments, then fall asleep. After it is asleep, place it back in the nest.

The baby will begin to stay awake for longer periods of time once the eyes are open. When this happens, it will be more fascinating to play with and to observe. As with any baby, it will require frequent naps and rest periods. But it will also require large doses of attention and love.

A baby that receives gentle and affectionate handling will respond by becoming very tame. It will rarely bite or become frightened and is a real pleasure to have around. Let the baby sit with you while you are reading or watching television. It will crawl all over you, exploring and examining everything. Eventually it will select a warm, snug place in your lap or beside you in the chair and curl up and go to sleep. Enjoying your orphan baby in this way will cause no difficulty when the time comes to let it go free.

If Baby Bites

As a rule, babies do not bite. If your baby makes an attempt to do so, however, chances are you are doing something wrong. A wild animal cannot stand physical restraint. Petting is one thing, but to clutch a squirrel is to invite a bite. If you try forcibly to subdue a raccoon, bobcat, or fox, you risk not only being bitten or scratched but also losing a friend.

Recognize what is natural and normal for your wild creature. Do not try to impose on your baby what you consider to be socially acceptable behavior. Most animals are guided by strong instincts. To attempt to discourage a bobcat from chasing birds or a raccoon from chasing mice and bugs is to thwart those instinctive urges upon which their survival depends.

As these instinctive urges to chase and pursue become stronger, you can be sure that the time to offer freedom is drawing near.

SETTING YOUR ORPHAN FREE

Offering freedom does not mean that you simply turn your orphan loose. The baby must have time to get used to a new life. It must learn to adapt to the world outside. When your orphan can run, romp, climb, and play, it is time to start the gradual process that will lead to full freedom. Do not make the mistake of waiting for the baby to be an adult. This would be a mistake. Start while the baby is young and flexible in its habits and can still learn about the wide world outside.

First Step

Freedom is given gradually, not all at once. To begin with, take your baby outside for an hour each morning and afternoon. Stay with it for the first few times. Initially, the animal may be afraid of the outdoors, which is a new and strange place. The baby may cling to you and be unwilling to move away. Be patient, for on the second or third try, the baby begins to gain confidence and will begin to do a little exploring close by you. It may go off on its own for a short distance, then come running back to you as if afraid you are going to leave.

As the baby grows accustomed to the outdoors, you will notice that when it is inside it will spend more and more time looking outside or pacing restlessly. It is time to start letting the baby go out on its own.

Second Step

Arrange for the door to be propped open at all times. This will allow the baby to come and go as it pleases, and, most importantly, give it ready access to its cage and nest box. Without a haven to escape to, the baby may be threatened and chased by animals that feel they own the territory around your house. The baby must find its place among the other animals in the area. But until it learns how to "fit in" and make its way among them, it must have the security of its own cage.

Before you know it, your baby will be out most of the time, coming in only for food once or twice a day, and at night to sleep in its nest home. When this happens, move the cage and nest home outside, placing it near the entrance the baby is accustomed to using, so your orphan can find it easily.

The half-grown baby, as it comes and goes, will still be glad to see you. It will like to be picked up and petted by members of the family. While it enjoys its freedom, it has not yet cut the ties with its human friends.

Then, one night, you will notice that the baby is missing, that it hasn't come back to the cage to sleep. You will worry and wonder if it is safe. Just remind yourself that the baby has learned to adapt to the outdoors and that this is another stage in your orphan's development. It is becoming a wild creature again.

Freedom

The cage will be used less and less often over the next weeks. Food will go uneaten. Several months later, the cage and house will be almost totally unused. Food is untouched. You may now and then see a familiar shape around your yard, but you will not be able to touch or handle it any longer. Your orphan has taken its place in nature, where it belongs.

To attempt to hold an orphan captive when it reaches maturity is cruel. It can also be dangerous. Deprived of its instinctive need to be with other animals of its kind, your former baby often becomes cantankerous. Even the handling of routine care can lead to a serious bite or scratch. There is no enjoyment in keeping an unhappy captive that cannot be handled. Nor can you even allow it to be set free. It will be too old to learn how to live successfully in the wild. The great satisfaction is in raising your orphan, in seeing it prepare itself to return to the wild, and in setting it free.

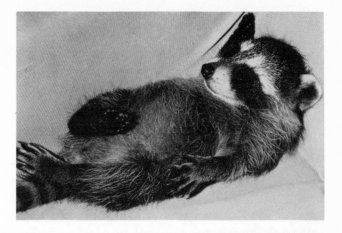

4

Ailing or Injured Mammals

INTESTINAL INFECTION

The most common infection in an orphan animal is an intestinal infection. This usually results from improper cleaning and care of the feeding utensils. The first sign of intestinal infection is a change in the baby's bowel material.

Normally, the bowel material will be slightly darker in color than egg yolk and about the consistency of toothpaste. If an infection is starting, the bowel material will appear at first slightly softer than usual and have little foamy bubbles. In the next stage, it will be more foamy and will look like thin formula, both in consistency and color. When this happens, you should start administering antibiotics.

Antibiotics

Antibiotics prevent or stop infection by killing or preventing the growth of disease-producing bacteria. Except in the case of baby rabbits, antibiotics are used only when an infection is present. Baby rabbits seem to be extremely sensitive to intestinal infection; therefore, as stated earlier, you may add antibiotics to their formula daily once their eyes are open as a preventative measure.

When you notice that the bowel material has become watery or loose, start administering antibiotics right away. Antibiotics are prescription items, so you will have to obtain these from your veterinarian. If you cannot see him personally, perhaps you can do it all by phone. Call him and explain your problem. Ask him if he can call in a prescription to your local drugstore.

One effective antibiotic in most intestinal infections is tetracycline. The usual daily therapeutic dose (the amount of antibiotic that must be given to kill or inhibit growth of disease-producing bacteria) is 50 milligrams (mg.) of tetracycline for each pound your patient weighs. Since most orphans are quite small, you will be dealing with ounces, not with pounds. Weigh the baby on a postal scale or kitchen scale. Use a daily dosage of 3 mg. of antibiotic for each ounce the baby weighs.

For example, a 2-ounce baby should receive 6 mg. of antibiotic, a 3-ounce baby should receive 9 mg., and a 4-ounce baby should get 12 mg. of this antibiotic each day.

To prepare the medication, dissolve one 250-mg. tetracycline capsule in 8 ounces of formula. Eight ounces is 240 milliliters, since each ounce is equal to 30 ml. Each milliliter of this formula thus contains 1 mg. of the antibiotic. If you feed this formula to your baby as you normally would feed plain formula, your baby should receive a satisfactory dosage.

The usual medicine dropper delivers ½ ml. to the baby each time. The average 2-ounce baby will take 12 dropperfuls of formula per day. The total amount of formula consumed is 6 ml. of formula and thus 6 mg. of antibiotic, the correct dosage.

However, your baby may take more or less than the average baby. Therefore, you must make sure it is getting the correct dosage. Calculate how much antibiotic the baby is actually receiving by counting how many dropperfuls it eats daily, divide by two to find out how many milliliters of formula it is taking and thus how many milligrams of antibiotic it is receiving. If the amount is not reasonably close, make an adjustment in the amount of antibiotic you are adding to the formula.

If the baby is not getting enough antibiotic in the formula consumed, add part of the contents of another capsule to the formula. It it is getting too much antibiotic, discard that formula, and mix up a new batch using only a portion of the capsule in your formula.

For smaller babies, add one capsule to their more concentrated 6-ounce formula. There will be slightly more antibiotic per milliliter or formula (1.4 mg. per milliliter), but since these babies consume less formula for their weight, the dosage works out right for them also.

Give the antibiotic until bowel eliminations return to normal and then for two additional days to be sure the infection is cleared up.

One point must be made very clear. Because in time of need a little antibiotic in the formula is good, that doesn't mean a lot is better. Too much antibiotic will reduce the baby's appetite so that it won't eat properly. So follow the guidelines and do not exceed recommended dosages.

DEHYDRATION

Sometimes intestinal infection can lead to dehydration. The formula may move through the intestinal tract so rapidly that the baby doesn't have a chance to digest and absorb the needed nutrients. The intestine becomes irritated. It loses water instead of absorbing it, and the baby becomes dehydrated (drying out from lack of water). Its skin feels dry instead of soft and pliable. Dehydration can progress so rapidly that after twelve hours, a fold of skin picked up between your thumb and fingers and then released may remain standing in a ridge. At this stage your baby will no longer eat. Death will follow shortly. The injection of fluids may save the orphan, but this can properly be done only by a veterinarian.

Sometimes, in spite of all you do, you will not be able to save your orphan. Knowing this can happen does not make it any easier to accept a death when it does occur. But if you do your best, you will have the satisfaction of knowing that you tried, and this is what is all-important.

TICKS, FLEAS, AND LICE

Most new babies you find will be neat and clean, but occasionally one may have fleas, ticks, or lice. In a very young baby with little or no hair, any parasite can be easily seen on the pink skin and removed.

Ticks are tiny, brownish, oval creatures which resemble spiders. They cling tightly to the skin by their mouth parts. You can pull them off with your fingers. Twist or rotate the tick in a clockwise direction as you pull gently, until it comes off.

Wrap the tick in a piece of toilet tissue and flush it down the toilet. Then wash your hands thoroughly with soap and water. Do not kill ticks by crushing them, since some contain disease-producing organisms.

Fleas and lice may not be as easy to spot. Fleas can be seen crawling rapidly through the hair if you check the baby's skin carefully. They are hard, shiny, slender, dark brown in color, and about the same size as the period at the end of this sentence.

Lice are usually slightly larger, soft, and a dull gray in color. They move slowly, if at all.

Treat fleas and lice in the same way. Use a flea spray which states on the label that it is safe for cats. Pyrethrins are generally the active ingredient.

Do not spray the baby directly. Spray into the palms of your hands, rub your hands together to disperse the fluid somewhat, and then rub it into the hair coat of your orphan baby. In this way the "hissing noise" of the spray can doesn't frighten the baby, and the insecticide will be evenly distributed over the entire body.

This spray is mild, so you may repeat the treatment the following day if necessary. If the baby looks grubby from flea dirt, bathe it.

BATHING

A baby may be bathed once, when you first adopt it, or occasionally if it has somehow soiled itself. But bathing should not be a regular weekly event. Most babies learn to clean and groom themselves.

You can bathe even the tiniest baby if you are careful. Adjust the water from the tap until it feels comfortably warm on your arm. Hold the baby gently in the palm of one hand, elevate the head end, so water won't get in its nose or mouth, and place the tail end under the gently flowing warm water.

With your other hand, massage water into the skin, rinsing the dirt away. Work toward the head end, cleaning as you go. Never put the head under the water. Clean the face with the tips of your moistened fingers.

If this rinsing isn't sufficient to clean the baby, use a mild soap, Johnson's Baby Shampoo, or even a mild dishwashing detergent. Lather the baby and rinse thoroughly.

The only real danger in this procedure is allowing the baby to become chilled. After the last rinse, wrap the baby in a towel and rub it gently until dry. Then hold it for a while so it can absorb the warmth of your hands, or place it back in its warm nest and cover it lightly with a piece of towel or some other soft material.

The baby will snuggle into your hands or into its nest and will be content to stay quiet until it is thoroughly dry and warm. Then it will usually become hungry.

Do not bathe the baby when it gets older. You might earn a bite or severe scratches from your usually docile orphan. No wild creature will tolerate being physically restrained, particularly if it becomes frightened.

INJURY

Should Help Be Given?

The first thing to determine is whether a creature really needs first aid. An abnormal physical appearance, abnormal behavior, and evidence of pain are signs that an animal, whether baby or adult, is in need of help.

ABNORMAL PHYSICAL APPEARANCE. An animal walking on three legs, or one with multiple wounds or with some part of its body swollen or enlarged, is one with an abnormal physical appearance.

ABNORMAL BEHAVIOR. A squirrel crawling slowly about in the middle of a busy highway is one example of abnormal behavior. Other examples are a skunk that wanders into your yard in the daytime. Or an adult fox or raccoon that appears friendly and allows you to come close. Abnormal behavior may be a sign of rabies. Avoid these animals completely. Report them at once to the local wildlife officer, health department, or police.

PAIN. The presence of pain is often hard to detect. Even a veterinarian cannot always tell if an animal feels pain. An animal in pain is uneasy and restless. It usually has an anxious expression, but it seldom whines or cries. Often it will lick at the area where the pain is most intense.

When Not to Help

The care and treatment of the smaller animal with concussion is probably the only animal first aid you will be able to handle yourself. When a larger full-grown animal such as a raccoon, opossum, deer, or bobcat is injured or sick, it will usually seek a secluded spot. Such an animal is dangerous and must not be approached without professional assistance. It will bite, scratch, or strike out with its feet if it feels threatened. More important, an injured animal trying to flee will probably do even more damage to itself. You can help most by calling the office of the nearest wildlife officer or game warden and describing the condition and exact location of the animal. He can usually determine if it can be moved.

After an animal with large wounds, fractures, or similar injuries has received the professional care it needs, you may offer to give the animal the necessary nursing care.

How to Administer First Aid

Let's go back to the squirrel on the highway. Let us say that it was able to lift its head and move a bit, but that it would not stand. This animal has undoubtedly been hit by a car. Internal injuries are common when a small animal collides with something as massive as an automobile. Unfortunately most of them will die. Sometimes, however, the animal is merely stunned or has a concussion. If the brain damage is not severe, many of those animals will recover with good nursing care.

MOVING THE ANIMAL TO SAFETY. Without endangering yourself, remove the animal from the highway as quickly as possible. The easiest way to do this is to use a jacket or sweater to protect yourself. Place the jacket over the squirrel and gently slide your hands underneath it, keeping the jacket between your hands and the animal's body.

Once you have the animal cradled in your hands and covered with the jacket, carry it to a place where you can care for it. Place it in a comfortable cage, or even a cardboard box, and allow it to rest. Provide the animal with a dish of fresh water. Maintain the temperature in the box or cage at about 80° F. by using a 60-watt bulb for extra heat, if necessary. Warmth is very important in the treatment of shock.

Lightly stunned animals may recover in one hour or less and can be released as soon as they seem to be walking and moving normally.

If the animal moves feebly but can't walk, it is suffering from a more severe concussion. It may be a month or more before it can move well enough to be set free. Allow it complete rest for the first twenty-four hours.

FLUIDS. If the animal is not drinking water or is semiconscious, start dropper-feeding it water. While any animal can go without food for several days, without fluids dehydration occurs and death follows.

Place the animal on its side. Do not tip the head up, or the water will run down into the back part of the throat, causing the animal to cough or choke. Fill the dropper with water. Place the tip of the dropper between the animal's lips and allow a few drops of fluid to trickle onto and across the tongue. In many cases the fluid will stimulate your patient to start licking and swallowing. Keep up a steady, gentle, slow trickle as long as your patient keeps licking and swallowing. Then allow it to rest.

ADDING FORMULA. An hour later, try again, using the proper milk and egg yolk formula.

Continue to give water and formula alternately every few hours during the day until your patient is able to drink on its own. This often takes several days. When it can lift its head and is more aware of what is going on, offer formula in a small shallow dish or jar lid. Place the dish under its chin and encourage it to try to lap the formula.

An animal that can take formula or water will almost always recover. However, one that does not respond to your efforts and will not swallow may have severe brain damage. Ask the opinion of your veterinarian on its chances for survival.

If it appears to your veterinarian that the animal will never recover completely, euthanasia may be better than prolonging the animal's suffering.

Birds

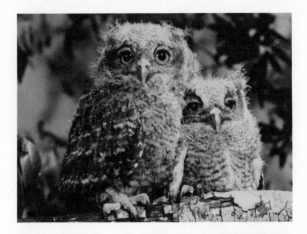

5

Altricial Birds

WHAT IS AN ALTRICIAL BIRD?

Altricial birds are born helpless. They are hatched in a weak condition and are, therefore, confined to the nest. Their eyes are usually still closed, and they have few or no feathers. They are completely dependent upon their parents for warmth and nourishment. All songbirds are altricial birds. So are woodpeckers, hawks, owls, crows, and many of the water birds, such as herons, egrets, and pelicans.

Because a baby altricial bird lives in the nest for several days to several months after hatching, it is called a nestling. From the time they leave the nest until they are independent of their parents, they are called fledglings.

WHAT IS AN ORPHAN?

An orphan is a baby bird without a nest or without parents. Many of the birds which need help are birds that leave the

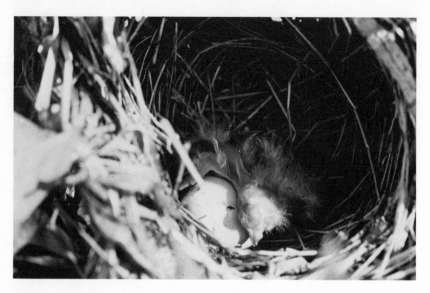

Nestling redwing blackbird, a helpless, blind, naked altricial bird.

nest prematurely. They either tried to fly before they were able, or they have fallen out. If you find a naked, helpless baby on the ground, try to locate its nest. It should be close by. If the baby bird seems warm and active, put it back in the nest at once. If it is trembling and appears cold, gently cup your hands around it until it feels warm, then place it back in the nest. If the nest has been destroyed or if you cannot find it, and if neither parent is anywhere nearby, the baby is an orphan. Adopt it.

Do not worry that because you have touched the baby its parents will abandon both it and the nest. There is truth to the belief that parent birds may desert the nest they are building if they are bothered. They may even do so during the first part of the incubation period. But they are not likely to do so once the eggs have hatched.

If you see the parents watching nearby, it is usually safe to leave the baby on a branch near the nest. They will feed and care for it as if it were in the nest. But if the baby persists in flying to the ground, where it faces constant danger, and you cannot see its parents, the baby is an orphan. Adopt it.

Determining Baby's Age

Since the way these orphans react to you and the care you must give them depend on their age, it is well to have an idea of the baby's age. This can be determined by several factors, but feathering and the presence of an egg tooth are the most important. The egg tooth is a small whitish projection near the tip of the upper beak, which the nestling uses to crack through the shell of the egg when hatching. The tooth usually disappears about three days after birth. Therefore, a naked baby with the whitish egg tooth projecting from the tip of the upper beak is less than three days old.

The nestling one week old or younger will be almost naked,

The egg tooth is the tiny, white projection near the tip of the beak of the baby screech owl on the left. The second one, one or two days older, has already lost the egg tooth.

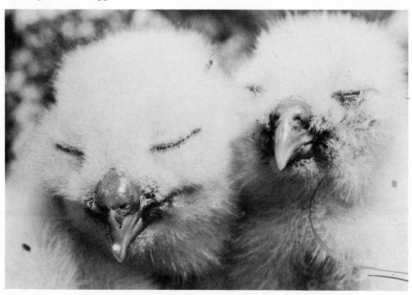

but will show some dark projections protruding from the skin. These projections, called pinfeathers, will emerge as feathers over the next two weeks. Feathers will first appear along the back and head, then on the wings, and finally on the abdomen and breast area. By two weeks of age, songbird babies have feathers covering most of their skin. By three weeks of age, most songbirds are well covered with feathers and are fluttering about, but not really flying. At four to six weeks of age, they can fly quite well.

Putting Baby Back in the Nest

FOR MOST BIRDS. The tiny altricial bird with only a few or no feathers can be easily picked up. Gently cup the baby in the palms of your hands. It will seldom flutter or struggle and will snuggle down to absorb the warmth of your hands. Usually an alert beady eye will watch you intently, as if to judge whether you are friend or foe.

Baby mockingbird is content being carried in hand-nest.

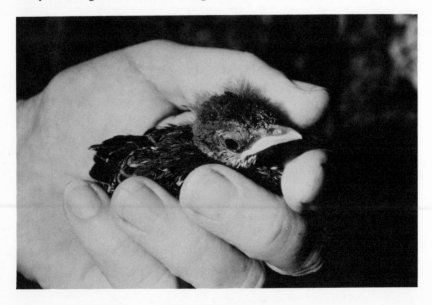

If the baby you have found is at the stage when it is almost ready to leave the nest, as evidenced by the fact that it has feathers all over, it will be extremely difficult to return this baby to its nest. It is so afraid of you that each time you release it at the nest, it will usually flutter away trying to escape.

A young nestling that has enough feathers to flutter away on short flights is more difficult to catch. Follow it slowly, herding it into the corner of a fence or a building, or into tall grass. Talk gently as you quietly approach. Usually, you will be able to trap the young bird in your hands. Once captured, it will usually sit quietly. However, a sudden movement or noise may frighten it, and it will flutter away again. So confine the baby gently but firmly enough in your hands to keep it from flying away, but don't squeeze it. Then return it to the nest.

FOR OWLS AND HAWKS. The baby owl or hawk doesn't usually use its sharp beak and claws for defense. If the baby is tiny and downy, pick it up in your hands and return it to its nest. If it is old enough to have some feathers, use a short stick or your fingers as a perch. Gently press the stick or finger against its abdomen. It will usually step on the perch rather than allow itself to be pushed backward. You may have to make as many as ten attempts. But once the bird is securely on the perch, you can carry it to the nest tree. If you can't find the nest, carry it on your finger or the twig perch to your home, where you can properly care for it.

WARMTH AND SHELTER

The Nest

The altricial orphan bird you have adopted must be provided with warmth and a nest. Use a box about 6 inches square as a nest. A quart berry basket will do nicely. Mold a

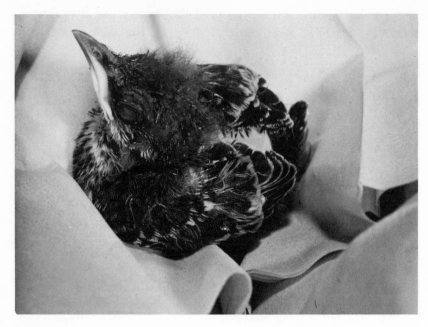

Mockingbird in nest made from berry box, lined with tissues.

soft piece of cloth, part of an old towel or flannel shirt, into a nest shape and place it inside the box. Then cover the whole nest with fifteen or twenty Kleenex-type tissues. Pat them down to assume a nest shape. The tissues will be used as disposable nest liners. Whenever the baby soils the nest, lift the soiled top tissue out, leaving a fresh one in position. When all the tissues are gone, put in a new stack.

Not all birds require a lot of clean-up care. You may even find a baby orphan that is partially toilet-trained. We raised a tiny bluejay only a few days old whose nest area never needed changing. Each time it felt the need to evacuate, it climbed to the edge of the nest, turned around, backed up close to the edge, and then with several ludicrous wiggles of its sparsely pinfeathered tail, evacuated its droppings well out of the nest area. While this is normal behavior in older nestlings, it is unusual in one so young.

Temperature Control

Provide warmth in the same way as for mammal orphans. Place the nest area away from cold drafts, and use a 60- to 100-watt bulb to provide heat. Place an inexpensive thermometer in the nest and move the light bulb closer and farther away from the nest until a nest temperature of 95° F. is consistently maintained. This temperature is correct for the very young bird with few or no feathers. Allow the bulb to burn night and day to provide constant warmth.

The normal body temperature of most altricial birds is about 102° F. or higher. Although our nest temperature is lower, the bird will receive enough radiant warmth to protect it. Too much heat can cause more harm than too little. A bird begins to acquire the ability to control its body temperature at about the time its feathers start to emerge from the protective sheaths or to change from pinfeathers. This is about midpoint in its nest life.

When the bird is fairly well covered with feathers, begin dropping the nest temperature by moving the bulb farther away from the nest. Decrease the temperature 5° F. each week until it reaches 70° F. Keep the light available as long as the bird sits near it and uses its warmth. Remove the light when the orphan is well feathered and sleeps in another part of the cage.

A baby bird less than a week or two of age will stay in its nest. When it perches on the edge of the nest and becomes more active, it is time to transfer the nest and light to a cage.

The Cage

Build the cage of hardware cloth, as discussed in Chapter 1. The size of the cage will vary a great deal depending on the size the nestling will be when full-grown. All cages should be at least 30″ × 30″ × 36″. This minimum size is adequate if the nestling when full-grown will be the size of a bluejay,

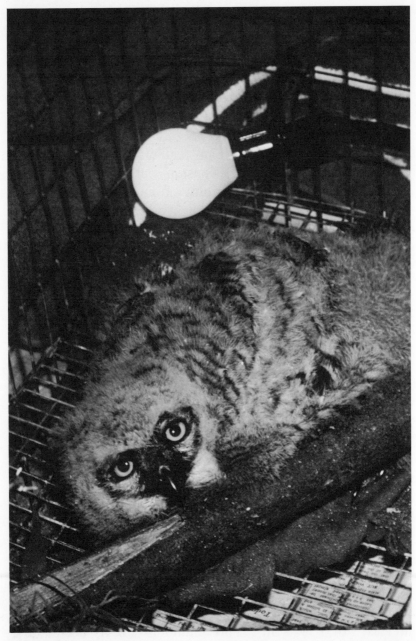

Great horned owl baby in cage with light bulb, nest area, and a perch.

mockingbird, or robin. Wire the nest, in its berry box, in one corner of the cage, about halfway up the side walls. Wire the thermometer in place at the edge of the nest box and the light bulb and socket against the outside of the cage at the same distance from the nest box as it was previously.

Having the bulb outside the cage makes for greater safety for an active, growing nestling, and allows the nest temperature to remain constant. When the orphan hops and flutters about the cage, there is no chance that it will land on the bulb and burn its feet.

Place perches of various sizes in the cage. Dead limbs trimmed from a tree and cut to the correct length are more suitable than smooth, polished perches, since rough bark gives the fledgling a better foothold. Vary the diameter of the limbs to keep the nestling's feet from becoming sore. In a cage 30″ × 30″ × 36″, wire five or six perches at various heights throughout the cage. Design it as you would a playground, with some jumping distance and others flying distance apart. Jumping and flying from perch to perch will help improve the fledgling's coordination.

Cover the bottom of the cage with several layers of newspaper to absorb moisture and help keep the cage clean. Change them about every other day.

We usually leave the cage door open during the day and allow the fledglings the freedom of a screened porch. They flutter and fly around the porch exploring, strengthening flight muscles, and improving coordination. They regularly return to the cage for food, rest, and warmth. When two or three birds are on a porch at once, there can be some confusion. Many birds are very antagonistic toward others on "their" porch. Often, but not always, a larger bird will pick on a smaller one. A tiny titmouse we had adopted would fly into the nest area of three young screech owls and take on all three at once. They had to be rescued from its fierce bites. From then on, we opened the two cages at separate times for the flying exercise periods. For the fledgling or nestling, cages represent security as well as confinement.

FEEDING MOST BABY BIRDS

Eating is one of the first activities a newly hatched altricial bird can perform. When first hatched, any noise or vibration which arouses it will cause the baby instinctively to raise its head and open its mouth wide to receive food. This is called "gaping."

To feed the very young bird, whose eyes are closed and whose egg tooth is still present, tap the side of the nest box gently as you prepare to offer it food. If the baby is healthy, it will gape—lift its head and open its mouth wide. When its beak is open wide, place food in the back part of its mouth.

Young mockingbird gapes for food.

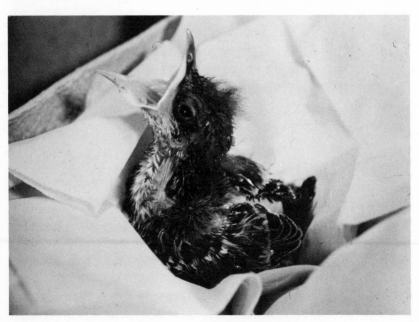

If it is so weak that it does not gape, then forced feeding will be necessary. This will be discussed later in the book, in the chapter on special feeding.

As the nestling learns to eat, it also learns to respond to visual stimulation. At three to four days of age it will open its mouth and gape when it sees your hand approaching the nest. At this time it is no longer necessary to tap or gently shake the nest box before offering each bite of food.

After the nestling is a week old, it will recognize you as an individual. When it is hungry and sees you approaching, it will stand up in the nest, flutter its wings rapidly, and cheep repeatedly as if to say "hurry, hurry, hurry!" This is called "begging posturing" and such behavior is a sign your orphan is maturing. Now it begins to develop "personality" and is the most fun to take care of.

If the bird you have found and adopted is already a week old, it will be shy. It will take patience and gentleness to get it to start eating. However, three or four days after it starts eating, it will accept you as a friend and show this welcoming behavior.

Once the nestling starts begging, lift it out of the nest at each feeding, place it on a perch at about the same distance from the bulb that the nest was, and feed it. Then return it to its warm nest.

The Basic Diet

Basically, the diet for all altricial birds, except doves, consists of bits of Purina Cat Chow moistened and softened in a formula of one egg yolk mixed into 6 ounces of homogenized milk.

Allow the hard dry pieces of cat chow to soak in a small amount of formula until they absorb enough moisture to make them soft. As they absorb moisture, the dry food swells. Each piece of cat chow will make two to four bite-sized pieces. The

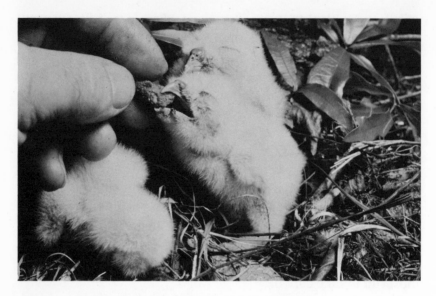

Baby screech owl accepting a bite-sized pellet of food.

bite-sized bits should not be so mushy that they lose their shape, but just be soft enough to be swallowed easily by the baby bird.

While the cat chow bits may also be moistened in water, the formula supplies additional high-quality nutrients to the bird's diet.

Discard the bits and pieces that aren't eaten, and prepare a few fresh bits for each feeding.

Feed the baby a bit of the moistened food, about the size of a pea. When the baby gapes, stuff the pellet into the back part of its throat. If you have ever watched a mother bird feed her young you know she is not gentle in the feeding process, but just pokes the food down the nestling's throat. But you should be gentle. If necessary, use your little finger to push the pellet partway down the throat—gently. If you don't place the food well back in the throat, the baby will spit it out.

Properly placed, the pellet will be swallowed at once. The small day-old bird may want to accept only one pellet. You can tap the nest box and move your hand toward its mouth to see if it might want more, but the smaller bird will not want any more food for thirty minutes to an hour, or even longer. A bird the size of a week-old blue jay will probably take four to six pellets, but it won't want to eat again for an hour or two.

Overfeeding is not usually a problem, since the babies stop eating when they have had enough. After a few days you will be able to anticipate when your bird will be ready to eat again.

As the baby bird gets older it will eat a little more at each feeding, and the interval between feedings will stretch to two or three hours.

Liquids

The moistened pellet of cat chow usually contains enough liquid to satisfy most babies. However, offer additional water several times a day and see if your baby desires it.

To offer the water dip a finger into a glass of clear, clean water. Usually one large drop will hang from the end of your finger. When the baby gapes, place your finger within reach of the baby. The bird will capture the drop off your finger. If it looks expectantly at you, offer water several more times until it refuses to gape.

Offer water in this fashion only after the baby has satisfied its hunger. Offering water when the nestling is hungry may make you mistake its apparent interest in your finger and water for thirst, when all it really wants is to eat.

When the nestling is older, place a water dish close beside the nest.

Feeding Doves and Dove-type Birds

Baby doves are quite different from other altricial birds. They are normally fed a liquid secretion regurgitated from the crop of adult birds. As orphans, they do not gape, but when they are hungry they poke and probe at your fingers with their bills, seeking food.

Since their normal diet is liquid in form, feed them a suitable semi-liquid food replacement in a way they can handle it.

The diet of a young nestling can be prepared by mixing cooked Wheatena or Ralston with an equal amount of human infant soybean milk formula powder, such as Similac or Mulsoy. The cereal and baby milk formula is diluted with water to make a thick soup. Make the formula thinner for a very young bird and thicker as it grows older.*

Since the baby dove normally feeds by inserting its bill in the parent bird's mouth and throat, offer the formula you have prepared in a similar fashion. The easiest way to do this is to remove the rubber bulb from a medicine dropper, or cut off the end of a nipple, and place your formula in this soft, pliable container.

Offer the open end of the rubber container to the baby. It will insert its beak to the nostrils and suck up the formula. You may gently compress the bulb or nipple to squeeze the formula toward the open end so the baby can get at it.

Refill the container and feed the baby until it is satisfied. Offer additional formula in an hour. You will soon learn how frequently and how much your orphan dove wishes to eat.

As the baby gets larger and grows nicely, place grit, bird grain, and water conveniently in the bottom of the cage. By the time it is feathered, the baby should be eating well.

Expanding the Menu

As the nestling gets older and begins hopping from perch to perch, offer it a variety of foods. Place some on the cage floor, others in small feeders wired to the perches, and still others fastened to the sides of the cage.

Read about your specific bird in a good bird book. For example, the National Geographic Society book *Song and Garden Birds of North America* is an excellent source of this information. It gives a picture of each bird, a brief description

* Formula courtesy of Pam Stewart, Bradenton, FL.

of its habits, and information on the bird's usual food. Try to offer some of the foods your bird would eat if it were free. Offer as great a variety as possible and allow the bird to choose what it wants.

Wild bird grain or a seed mixture is essential for seed eaters and will be eaten by many other birds. It is available in grocery stores, pet shops and feedstores. Also provide breakfast cereals, brown bread crumbs, fruits such as grapes, sections of oranges, and apples, and vegetables such as bits of celery, carrots, and lettuce for your birds to try. Bits of eggshell or oystershell should also be offered. They are an excellent source of calcium, and oystershell will help the bird digest its food. Oystershell may be obtained at any livestock feedstore in a rural area or a pet shop in the city.

Since birds have no teeth, most of the food is ground up in the gizzard after it has been swallowed. This heavily muscled organ squeezes food and seeds together rhythmically, breaking them into very small pieces, which then pass into the intestine. Hard materials such as oystershell, called grit, stay in the gizzard and function as a grinding agent to break up the seeds and bits of food. Eventually grit is worn down and the bird eats more to replace it. Your orphan may not eat much oystershell with the diet you are feeding. It is not an absolute necessity, since the cat chow contains extra calcium and is easily digested.

As your bird eats more and more of the foods you supply, you will begin to notice which food it likes best. Continue to feed the cat chow "baby-style" as long as the bird wants it, but less and less frequently. Soon the fledgling will eat adequately on its own. However, many birds seem to enjoy being fed, so continue hand-feeding your fledgling two or three times a day as long as it wishes.

Many of our birds that are adult in appearance still fly to us and expect to be hand-fed for several months after they are capable of finding food on their own. Other birds are more independent and wean themselves almost at once.

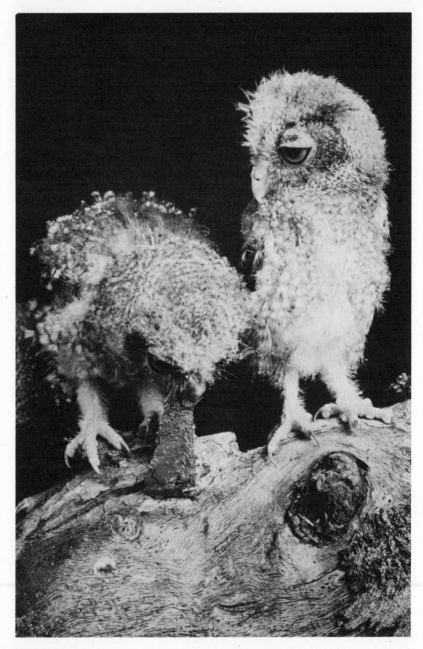

Baby screech owl eats a piece of beef heart.

FEEDING HAWKS AND OWLS

Hawks and owls are also altricial birds, but because they are predators they require special care. They normally live by capturing small animals such as mice and rabbits. Although basically meat eaters, along with the muscle or meat of their victim the hawks and owls also eat the skin, stomach contents, internal glands, and sometimes even fur and feathers. Thus, in the wild, they actually eat a variety of substances, not just meat. The digested portion of the prey provides a balanced diet. The undigested material such as bones, hair, fur, or feathers is usually regurgitated (spit up) as a round ball or "pellet" some twelve hours after eating.

When very young, hawks and owls gape just as other birds do. Feed the very young baby birds cat chow moistened with egg and milk formula just as you would songbirds. Give them as much as they want to eat four to six times daily. When they have eaten enough, they will refuse to accept more. Each bird seems to establish its own eating pattern.

When hawk and owl babies are two weeks old, feed them four times daily. While owls normally eat at night, with the light bulb burning all the time there will be no night or day, and they will eat whenever you offer food.

When you see feathers showing through the down, it is time to offer them strips of beef heart at every other feeding. Alternate the moistened cat chow feeding and beef heart until the baby is eating the beef heart well. You can obtain beef heart at most supermarkets or butcher shops. Cut it into pieces about 2 by 4 by 4 inches in size, wrap each piece individually, and store it in the freezer. Thaw one piece at a time as needed.

Cut the piece into strips about ¼ inch thick. At first, offer tiny bite-sized bits to the nestling. Once it eats a piece or two, it will like both the flavor and consistency. As it gets a little older and eats more readily, offer larger pieces so it will learn to tear and play with the meat. At this time add supplements to the beef heart to make it a balanced food.

Dip the meat strips in egg yolk, which will increase the fat content and add additional vitamins, then powder it lightly with a calcium-vitamin-mineral supplement. Since most birds only have from forty to one hundred taste buds in the back part of their mouths (as compared to nine thousand in man), you will have little difficulty getting your bird to accept the meat coated with the rather bland calcium supplement.

Make the powdered supplement by combining equal parts of calcium carbonate powder and a good veterinary vitamin-mineral supplement. Any drugstore has or can get the calcium carbonate powder for you, and your veterinarian will supply you with an appropriate vitamin-mineral supplement. This is the only time we use a vitamin-mineral supplement in our feeding program.

When your hawk or owl baby reaches the age where it is beginning to fly, discontinue the canned cat chow altogether and use only the basic beef heart supplement diet.

Offer the beef in larger slices, about 3 inches long and ½ inch thick, so the fledgling will learn to grasp it in its talons and use its sharp beak to tear it into bite-size portions. It must learn to do this with food if it is to survive in the wild.

Offer fresh road-killed birds and small animals for the same reason. It is a necessary part of their training for them to eat creatures they might prey upon in the wild. We do not, however, offer them live animals as food.

Provide fresh water at all times for all hawks and owls, regardless of their age.

Several at a Time

If you are caring for several birds of prey at one time, it is easier to buy a prepared diet. Zu-Preem Bird of Prey Diet, prepared by Riviana Foods, Inc. (Hills Division, Topeka,

Kansas 66601), is an excellent food used by many zoos. However, 32 pounds is the smallest package size available, and most distributors will not deliver orders of less than 200 pounds. Unless you live in a city with a distribution center that will allow you to pick up one case at a time, or unless you can pool your order with other people, it will not be practical to use this product.

Most birds will accept the Zu-Preem diet well, but they seem to prefer the beef heart supplement diet. For those caring for only one or two birds at a time, the beef heart supplement diet has the advantage of always being available, although it is certainly not any less expensive. We have maintained hawks and owls that could not be freed because of permanent injuries on the beef heart supplement diet for several years. They were healthy, active, and bright, with no sign of dietary deficiency.

Many publications state that it is necessary to feed fur, feathers, and bones to hawks and owls, so that they can properly digest their food. This is not so. We have maintained owls and kestrels for years without ever feeding them a single bone, feather, or bit of fur.

HANDLING AND FREEDOM

You cannot hold, handle, and caress a wild bird as you would a mammal baby. When tiny, birds seem to enjoy being held in a nest of your cupped palms. But they do not enjoy being petted or cuddled.

However, they do enjoy being talked to, and while keeping you company, they will snuggle down to enjoy the warmth that radiates from your body. When the nestling becomes a fledgling, it will enjoy sitting on your finger, riding around on your shoulder, even sleeping on your shoulder. The more time you spend with it, the more tame it will be and the more it will seem to enjoy your company. It flies to you for companionship and food.

If you obtain a bird when it is very small, it will be "imprinted" on you and your family. This means you are its parents and its world. When it is fully feathered and can fly well, you cannot just turn it loose one morning and expect it to survive. It will want to be with you and will fly to you for attention and companionship. This transition to freedom is a gradual process, regardless of species.

Freeing Most Birds

When you notice the fledgling no longer uses the nest or seeks the warmth of the light, it is time to start planning for its eventual release and freedom. Remove the light and place the cage on a screened porch or in some similar place, where the fledgling can see and hear other birds outside. Leave the cage door open whenever possible, so it can practice flying. You will notice it listens attentively to other birds and begins chirping and "singing" when it reaches three to four weeks of age.

At this stage, take the fledgling outdoors for "flying lessons." At first it will appear to be afraid. It may fly to a nearby tree for a moment and then fly back to you. It will hop about the grass exploring, but, unless frightened away, will stay close to you. Start with flying lessons for twenty- to thirty-minute periods twice daily. After three or four days, your orphan will spend more time away from you. It may enjoy being left alone for short periods while you return to the house. But when you go outdoors again, after it has been alone, it will fly to you the minute it sees you. As you start into the house, if it is not ready to go in, it will fly back into a tree. If it has had enough exercise and is hungry, the fledgling will sit on your hand or shoulder for the ride inside to its cage.

If it doesn't come to you, leave it and return in a half hour to try again. We have never had a bird get lost or leave us until it has had many outdoor sessions and has adapted to freedom.

The periods outside will become longer and longer by the fledgling's own choice, but it will still want the security of its cage at night. If you have a screened porch, place its cage where it is safe from cats, and prop the porch door partially open so it can come and go as it pleases. If you have no porch, hang the cage under the eaves where it will have some protection from wind and rain, beside the door you usually use. Keep food and water in the cage, and the bird will use it regularly.

One night you will notice that your bird did not come to the cage. This is a sign your fledgling is growing up. You can place a piece of red or yellow plastic tape loosely on one leg just above the foot to distinguish your orphan from the neighborhood birds. This will wear off in time, but when you see the tape you will know your fledgling is in the yard and that it is all right.

Young hawks are offered freedom in the same fashion as the other altricial birds. They will instinctively try to catch small moving objects. Food is offered and kept available until they learn to capture their own. They gradually adapt to the world and spend less time near their cage.

Freeing Owls

Young owls are more active at dusk and early evening, so they must be given their freedom differently. When owl babies can fly well, move their cage outdoors where it has some protection from wind and rain. Allow them a few days to get acclimated, then start leaving the cage door open in the evening. During the night they will leave the cage and fly about, but usually they will be in their cage in the morning. Even those that prefer to "roost" in a nearby tree will come back each evening for food.

Hand-raised baby owls come to know your voice and will answer when you call. When they are first given their freedom, they will stay close to the house in nearby trees. If you walk under the trees at dusk, calling for your young owl, it will "squeak" an answer to you. Each time you call, listen quietly for a moment. The answer is not very loud, so you have to be fairly close to hear it. Sometimes when you call, the young owl will fly directly to you. If it does, offer it food in or near its cage. If it won't come to you, place food where it can see it and also place some in the cage.

Baby owls must be fed and have food available while they teach themselves to hunt. You may have to feed some fledglings each evening for several months, while others refuse your offerings much sooner. When the fresh food you place near or in the cage each night is not touched for three to four weeks, you can assume your youngster no longer needs your help.

Usually orphans raised with much love and attention stay tame for the first year, but after they migrate or go through a nesting season they become wild creatures again.

We know very well that helping a single bird isn't going to affect the overall ecosystem of the area, but in our family the joy of helping an orphan is satisfaction in itself. The enjoyment of raising it, of seeing this bit of life mature and return, flying, to its own environment, and of recognizing its individual flash of color in the yard is reward in full for a small amount of effort.

6

Precocial Birds

WHAT IS A PRECOCIAL BIRD?

Unlike altricial birds, precocial birds are much more independent when they are hatched. Their eyes are open when they hatch and within minutes they can stand and walk. They are covered with down, and their first feathers begin to appear within five to six days. Precocial birds usually remain in the nest for only a few hours, a day at the most. They may be partially dependent on their parents for food or may have to be taught to eat, but most of them begin immediately searching for food. The downy young of the precocial birds, which are usually called chicks, include killdeer, quail, pheasant, and turkey. But many water birds, including coots, ducks, and geese, are also precocial birds.

With such great differences between altricial birds and precocial birds, the care required varies considerably.

THE ORPHAN

Since precocial baby birds have been taught to eat and find their own food by the time they are two or three days old, they seldom need help. But things might go wrong in very cold or wet weather. The body temperature control mechanism of a chick does not function well until it is about four weeks old. The young chick huddles under its mother for warmth at night, or if it gets chilled. If the chick gets wet, chilling is a distinct possibility if it gets separated from the mother bird, for the down loses its insulating value. A wet, cold chick requires help only until it is warm and dry. Simply placing it in a cardboard box and suspending a 60-watt bulb close to it to provide warmth for a few hours may be all the help it needs. When it is warm and dry, it should be released where you found it. If the mother bird is close by, the chick will call and she will come back as soon as you leave. You can watch from a vantage point to see if the mother returns. If she has not found the chick within three or four hours, it would be best to assume the mother bird's responsibility yourself. If you know the mother has been killed, the chick should be treated as an orphan and offered whatever care is needed until it is old enough to survive by itself.

APPROACHING THE ORPHAN

Chicks Less Than Three Days Old

All tiny birds, whether they are quail-type land birds or baby ducklings, should be approached quietly, while you talk gently to them. The baby three days of age or under will usually sit quietly and allow itself to be picked up in your hands without moving or struggling.

The problem with birds less than three days of age is not in capturing them, but in finding them. For example, a group of birds at the roadside whose mother has just been killed by a car will scatter into the roadside grass. They huddle into tiny, well-camouflaged balls of fluff, and it takes time and diligent searching through the grass to locate the chicks. As you find them, gently pick them up. If you have to carry several, place them in a box or covered basket, or loosen your shirt a little, making a pouch of the material that droops over your belt. This pouch offers warmth, security, and confinement without danger of crushing.

Chicks More Than Three Days Old

If the chicks are more than three to four days old, they will flee from you as you approach. You will have to herd them into a spot where they can't run, and then pick them up. If you find them along the roadside, herding them into the tall matted grass will often slow them down enough to allow you to capture them.

If they are quick and flutter about trying to flee, leave them be. You probably won't be able to capture them, and they stand a better chance of survival in a group than dispersed singly over the whole area. If they can run well and fly a little, they can also find their own food.

WARMTH AND SHELTER

As for altricial birds, two of the primary requirements are warmth and shelter.

Baby precocial birds should be placed in a cage. While birds less than three days old are docile and are not fearful, they can run. They will often try to escape if a noise or sudden movement frightens them and may injure themselves.

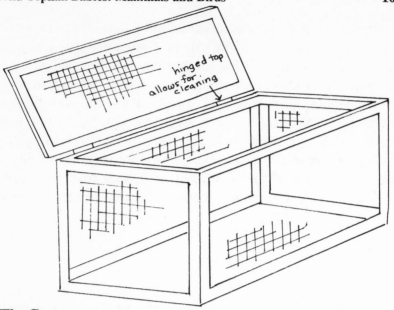

The Cage

A baby quail, pheasant, turkey, duck, or goose needs a cage 18″ × 24″ in size, with wire screen sides 12″ to 14″ high. This size would be suitable for several small baby chicks.

The cage sides should be made of hardware cloth or screen material to allow fresh air and light to enter.

It should have a removable top, to make it easy for you to clean, feed, and water your orphans. The cage may be constructed simply by tacking hardware cloth to a simple wood frame.

Place several layers of newspaper in the bottom of the completed cage to absorb water and droppings. Place a small pile of dried grass or shredded paper in one corner to serve as a nest area.

Provide water in a small shallow dish in another corner of the cage.

Put the cage in a draft-free area and place the baby or babies in it. Immediately provide the next essential item of care—warmth.

Warmth

For all precocial chicks use a brooding temperature of 95° F. Suspend a 60- or 100-watt bulb inside the cage in the corner near the nest. Place a thermometer on the floor of the cage under the bulb. As need be, raise or lower the light bulb about every ten minutes until the 95° F. is maintained on the thermometer. Leave the bulb in this position as long as the birds are in the cage. Be sure the bulb does not touch any of the paper or other materials which might burn.

Provide a sheltered corner near the light bulb. Cut a piece of cardboard the height of the sides and about 24 inches long. Fold it in half and tape it to the two adjoining walls. The cardboard will also serve to absorb heat from the bulb and radiate it on the baby when it seeks this spot for warmth and comfort.

The babies will move in and out of the warmth of the light bulb as they become warmer or cooler. Since they select the temperature they desire, you never have to change the position of the bulb. These birds also do not mind the brightness of the light and do not need periods of darkness for sleeping.

FEEDING

What to Feed

As food, offer a quail, pheasant, turkey, or other tiny, downy, seed-eating chick parakeet seed temporarily until a better food is purchased or prepared. Soaking the seed in water for five to ten minutes will make it more palatable.

If you live in a rural area that has a livestock feedstore, they will have a food called "chick starter" which is a finely ground combination of feed grains and vitamin and mineral supplements. If chick starter is not available in your area, make your own. Mix one third cup of dried bread crumbs with one hard-boiled egg yolk, and add sufficient milk to make a mass that will stick to itself but is dry enough to be rather crumbly. Feed it in bits about ⅛ inch in diameter. Chick starter or the homemade starter is suitable for ducks and other water birds, also.

When the birds are two to three weeks old and have more feathers, give them additional foods, such as lettuce, celery tops, or other green, leafy vegetables.

Check in the book already mentioned, *Song and Garden Birds of North America,* or the National Geographic Society companion volume *Water, Prey, and Game Birds of North America* for suggestions on the specific food your orphan would normally eat in the wild. If possible, offer whatever foods you can find that would be the same or similar to what the bird will feed on when it is free.

Teaching the Chick to Eat

Cover part of the floor near the bulb, or even the entire cage floor, with plain brown paper to provide the baby with a feeding area. Scatter the chick starter over the brown paper. It is important to make it as easy as possible for the chick to find its food. Newspaper does not work as well. Bits of food scattered on newspaper tend to confuse the chick. It often cannot distinguish between food and the letters and patterns on the newspaper. On clean brown paper, seeds and bits of food show up distinctly.

Place more food in a shallow dish or jar lid. You can use a chick feeder, a trough-type feeder which can be purchased at a livestock feedstore. This can be used by all precocial birds, including ducks and geese.

In the wild, a chick is taught to eat by the mother bird. Softly chirping or making the specific "food call," the mother bird will pick up a seed or other bit of food and drop it in front of the chick to attract its attention. The chick will usually pick

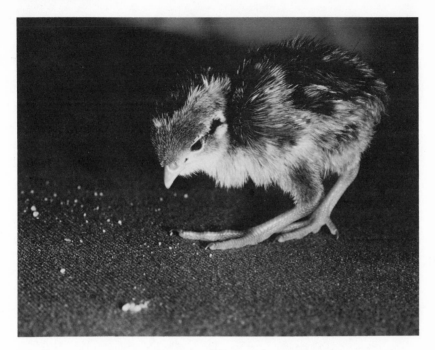

Bits of food scattered over a plain surface show up distinctly.

it up and swallow it. In this way, it learns to peck at bits and spots it sees on the ground.

The healthy chick will be interested in food as soon as it becomes warm and dry. If it doesn't pick at the food you offer, you must try the mother bird's feeding technique. Repeatedly drop bits of food in front of the chick to draw its attention to it. This must be done without frightening the chick, or it will flee to the far corner of the cage and will not be interested in food until it quiets down. When it appears to be moving about the cage exploring again, you know it is no longer frightened, and by talking quietly and gently to it, you can try feeding it once more, being "mother" again.

If you aren't certain your baby quail is eating, it is essential that you use the "toothpick" method of feeding (see Chapter 7) to ensure the life of your baby chick.

Feeding Ducklings, Geese, and Water Birds

Use a similar technique to get baby ducklings and other waterfowl to eat. Ducklings are used as the example, because they will be the most common water bird orphan found. Place bits of food in a shallow feeding dish or bird feeder. Scatter a few more bits around the floor of the cage. If they don't eat, here is a feeding method most ducks can't resist. Place a few bits of food in water in a dish with sides about 1 inch high. Straight-sided dishes are best, so the duckling can walk right up to the water and reach into it and feed without entering the water. It may anyway, but if it stays out, the water and food will stay cleaner. A baby duckling will drink the water, duck its head under the water, and playfully shake water everywhere. In playing, it will pick up and eat any little bits of food it sees in the water, or floating by. In general, if there is water it will make a mess, but that is part of being a duck— and as long as they start to eat, we don't mind.

SPECIAL HOUSING AND FEEDING

All precocial birds whether land birds or water birds are offered the same type of cages and foods until they are two to three weeks old. At this age they should be eating well, have some feathers, and be active and playful.

Because land and water birds are so different, the housing, care, and feeding procedures must be different from this point on.

Precocial Land Birds

Quail are the most common precocial birds which are raised as orphans. We will use them as our example, but the same housing, care, and feeding can apply to all land-type precocial birds whether they are pheasants, turkeys, grouse, chukars, or any other. The following applies to caring for several birds at one time.

HOUSING.   Precocial land birds must have more space than a small cage for exercise and more natural conditions if they are to adapt well to freedom. All land bird chicks should be transferred to a larger movable pen out of doors as soon as they begin to be well feathered. Construct a pen with a wooden frame about 4 feet square and 2 feet high, with sides of fine wire mesh or hardware cloth, but with no bottom. This will allow a natural outdoor environment of grass and weeds in the cage wherever it is set up. The pen must have a top to protect the chicks from predators. Wire one or two low perches in place at one end of the cage.

Place the outdoor pen in a grassy spot close to the house. Connect an extension cord to the same light you used in the smaller cage and place it in one corner of the new pen. Construct a three-sided shelter with a top, large enough to protect the light bulb from rain and to shelter your chicks from the cold, and place it in one corner of the cage. A shelter about 18

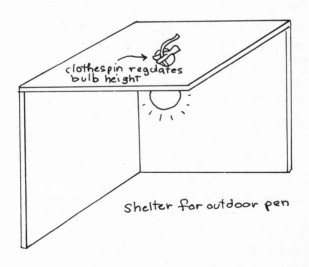

clothespin regulates bulb height

shelter for outdoor pen

inches square would be right for a group of smaller precocial birds, such as quail, or for one or two pheasant-size birds.

FEEDING. Use the same feeders and waterers as in the smaller cage. Offer the same food for the first few days to keep to a minimum changes which might upset the chicks. When the chicks are no longer frightened and are eating well, begin offering them wild bird grain mix, which consists of cracked corn, wheat, millet, sorghum grain seeds, and often sunflower seeds. It is sold in grocery stores or feedstores.

Offer both this feed and the chick starter in separate feeders and also scatter some in the grass, so the chicks will learn to "scratch" for food. They will instinctively use their feet to stir up the area between the grass roots as they carefully search about for edible bits of food and seeds. Move the pen as often as necessary to keep it clean and to offer a new variety of green plants.

Keep the chicks under these conditions until they are ready to be returned to the wild.

SETTING THEM FREE. Two factors will determine when the birds should be freed: weather and the amount of feathers. As has been said, a precocial chick's body temperature regulating mechanism is not completely functional until about four weeks of age. Since down and feathers act as insulation, the milder the temperature or the more feathers the chick has, the better the chick can survive without supplemental heat and the sooner it can be turned loose.

When you see that your chick no longer sleeps in the lamp-warmed area of the pen, but sleeps on one of the low perches you have provided at the other end of the cage or nestles in the grass elsewhere in the cage, unless colder weather has been forecast for the next few days, you can safely turn your chicks loose. Normally, chicks do not need to be kept past four weeks of age.

If adequate cover, such as heavy grass and bushy thickets, for their protection exists in the area around your home, release them there. Early in the morning open one corner of the cage slightly and allow the chicks to find the opening and to drift out.

Food is fairly abundant in late spring and early summer, and the chicks should have no trouble finding all they need. You may scatter food near the cage, or leave the cage open for several days, but these birds, when raised in a group, rarely return.

SETTING THE SINGLE BIRD FREE. The single bird that has been found and raised by itself will be very attached to you and must be allowed more time to adapt to freedom. Offer it its freedom as you would an altricial bird. Gradually allow it to spend more time outside. In time it will begin to prefer freedom to your companionship. Sooner or later it will find other wild birds and will drift away.

Precocial Water Birds

Ducklings are the most common precocial orphans you will have the occasion to raise. There is seldom a need to raise or rescue other precocial water birds, such as coots, gallinules, limpkins, rails, avocets, or the many others. The parents of these species are very shy and normally would not have their young where they would even be seen by humans. However, if any of these other species are found, housing and care would be the same as for orphan ducklings.

DIET. There would be slight changes in the diet of the different species. Comprehensive information on the subject can be obtained from reading *Water, Prey, and Game Birds of North America,* mentioned earlier. In the wild the various ducks feed on wild celery, a variety of grasses, shellfish and mollusks, pond weeds such as duckweed, aquatic insects, acorns, and the seeds of pond weeds and sedges. You may try to offer some of the foods, such as seeds, green succulent vegetation, grasses, and insects. However, the basic duckling diet which consists of chick starter, wild bird grain, lettuce, celery tops, and other green, leafy vegetables will provide the majority of water birds with the nutrients they need. Chick feeders or other feeding dishes should be provided for the chick starter and wild bird grain mixture. Those for which insects are an important part of their diet may be offered mealworms and earthworms in addition to this basic diet. Mealworms can be obtained at a pet shop and earthworms at a bait-fishing shop.

HOUSING.   As soon as baby ducks are eating well, place them in a 4′ × 4′ pen identical to the one used for land bird chicks. In addition to providing warmth and shelter, you must now also provide water for the babies to swim and play in.

Ducklings should have water to swim in as early as possible. If they are raised in a pen without water to swim in, they will be frightened of the water when you free them. If you force ducks that are afraid of the water into the water, they will come out as soon as you allow them to. In time they will adapt to the water, but this can take weeks, and all the time they stay on shore they are vulnerable to predators.

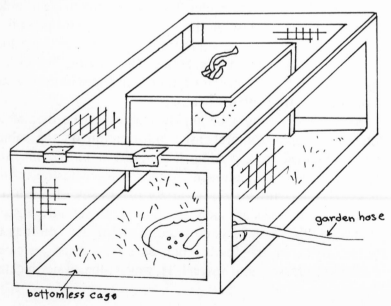

garden hose

bottomless cage

When baby ducklings are tiny, use an aluminum cake pan as a swimming pool. Place an inch of water in the pan and allow the babies to play in the water for ten or fifteen minutes twice daily. Young downy ducklings love the water. But they should not be permitted to stay in too long. Their down gets wet, they chill, and weak babies will die. They should be allowed to become acquainted with the water, and have the enjoyment of playing in it; but remove them before they get too wet or chilled.

As they get older they can have their swimming pool for longer periods of time. When they have some of their feathers and are ready to be moved to the larger outside pen, they can use the swimming pool as long as they like.

When we move our ducklings outdoors, it is easy for us to supply swimming water. We live on the edge of a lake in Florida where the temperature is quite warm during the spring, the "duckling" season. We place our pen in the sunshine, half in and half out of the water. The ducklings can enter and leave the water as they desire. Fresh water is constantly provided in the cage area, and bits of natural food are always floating by. Our ducklings can easily swim, play, and learn to eat.

Since we can't provide a light bulb at the lake shore we have to bring the ducklings back to the original, smaller cage at the house every night. On cold days they remain in the smaller cage, where their bulb is available for warmth, but most days they are outside at the lake shore.

If you don't have a lake, pond, or stream you can provide them with a swimming-playing area by digging a shallow hole to fit a large plastic dishpan. Place the dishpan in the ground so that its rim is at ground level. Build a ramp of stones or sand in one side so the ducks can walk in and out of their pool easily. Keep the pan full of water and maintain a constant supply and exchange of clean water by allowing a garden hose to trickle very slowly into the dishpan all day.

Place some of the wild bird mixture you are feeding the

chicks in the swimming pool as well. The ducklings will quickly learn to dive and feed off the bottom of the pool, which is the natural way for most ducks to feed.

If you live in a climate that is still cold in duckling season, you must provide your orphans with warmth in their pen. Suspend a 100-watt light bulb in the corner of the pen farthest from the swimming pond and protect it from splashing water. Make a wooden three-sided shelter in that corner to provide a warm, draft-free, protected corner for the ducklings and to protect the bulb further.

SETTING THEM FREE.   When it is time to set your ducklings free, do so where they can gradually become acclimated to being on their own. Most ducklings adapt to freedom easily and learn to find their own food readily, but some will need help and encouragement. By providing food grains, you can usually be sure the adaptation will be easy. Choose a place to free them where it will be convenient for you to feed them once a day. Scatter wild bird grain mixture in the shallow water and on the shore at the water's edge. This daily feeding gives you a chance to see how your youngsters are doing. Unless frightened away, young ducklings usually stay in the immediate area where you release them.

Two or more ducklings tend to keep one another company and adapt to freedom much more quickly. Since ducklings are capable of finding their own food at hatching, and are not extremely sensitive to cold temperatures, they can be offered freedom much earlier than most birds.

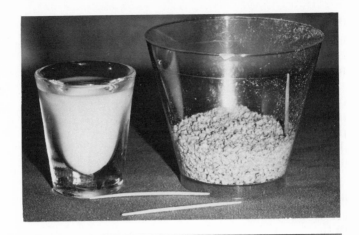

7

Feeding Injured
and Very Weak Birds
and
Dietary Supplements

TOOTHPICK FORMULA FEEDING

It can happen for one reason or another that a bird is too weak to eat. An altricial baby may be so weak it cannot gape, a precocial chick too exhausted to try to eat, and an injured bird may have no desire for food. These birds require special feeding techniques.

The weak altricial baby and the exhausted precocial chicks are fed in exactly the same way—by "toothpick formula feeding." However, be sure to warm the baby thoroughly before

115

offering it food. Follow the same warming procedures as described earlier. Take the concentrated formula as discussed
in Chapter 2 of one egg yolk in a half cup of homogenized
milk, and pour a small amount into a small glass or vial.

Cradle the baby in the fingers and palm of one hand in an
upright position. With your other hand, dip a flat, thin
toothpick into the formula. Hold the toothpick straight up and
down as you would a pen or pencil with the wide, flat end
downward. A small drop of formula will collect on the end
of the toothpick.

Touch this drop to the baby's beak near the tip. The upper
and lower beak meet here, and the liquid will flow into the
crack where the beaks meet. When most baby birds feel liquid
in their mouths, they will swallow.

If your bird is so weak that it doesn't swallow at once, tip
the baby forward slightly. This will keep the formula from
trickling down the throat by gravity, and will allow it to remain in the tip of the beak until it is swallowed.

Any gentle movement to make the baby aware of its surroundings, such as touching its beak with the toothpick or
gently moving your left hand to make the baby shift position,
will also help stimulate swallowing.

Even the tiniest quail baby will swallow drop after drop as
it is offered on the toothpick. When the baby no longer wants
more, it will refuse to swallow and instead will sling its head,
throwing the liquid from its beak.

That is the time to put the baby back in its nest, near the
light bulb, and allow it to rest. Try to feed it again thirty
minutes later. The baby will usually accept and swallow the
drops more readily at the second feeding. It may take twenty
or more drops this time.

When the baby has taken as much as its wants or as much
as it can handle, put the baby back in its nest and try again in
an hour. On this third feeding, the bird should open its beak,
reach out, grasp the end of the toothpick, and swallow the

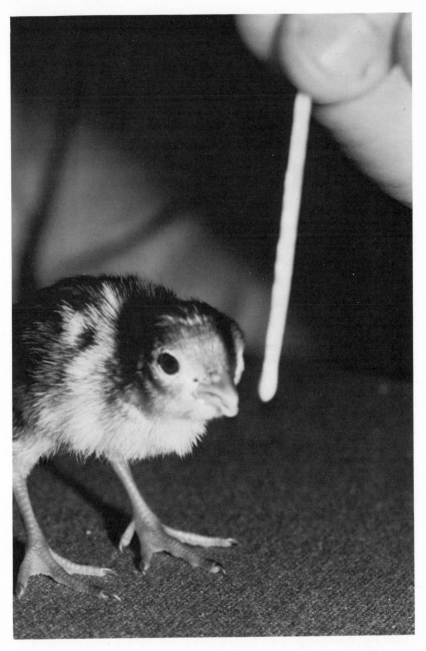

Too weak to eat, baby quail accepts formula from end of toothpick.

drop of formula. Feeding has now become an active process, with the orphan helping.

Each time you feed it, the general attitude and appearance of the bird will improve. If the weak, lethargic altricial bird will now gape, you may offer bits of moistened cat chow between each toothpick formula feeding. As the young precocial bird becomes stronger, it will be more interested in food, and will begin moving about pecking at bits in the feeding area.

You may have to use toothpick feeding only once or twice, or you may have to continue for several days. Stop when the orphan is eating other food well.

Most bird books insist that attempting to feed liquids to a bird will kill it. This is not so. The only thing to watch out for is that the bird is swallowing. If the bird is swallowing you have nothing to worry about. Swallowing is an active, voluntary process. The opening to the windpipe closes during this process. If the bird is not swallowing, the fluid may trickle down the throat by gravity and get into the windpipe and lungs. But there is no danger if you use common sense and good judgment when offering liquids.

Use an adaptation of the toothpick-feeding technique for sick or injured adult birds which have lost the desire to eat. You can feed them the same formula, but use a medicine dropper for larger birds instead of a toothpick.

Hold the bird upright. Keep the head tipped slightly downward, and trickle the fluid one drop at a time into the bird's beak until it will no longer swallow it.

STOMACH-TUBE FEEDING

If your bird is so weak that it can't be aroused, there isn't much hope for it. However, as a last resort, you can still try tube force-feeding. For the majority of birds, this will not be necessary.

The same equipment is used for birds as for orphan mammals (see p. 53), but the technique is simpler. Two people are needed for this procedure. Attach a small plastic syringe containing 1 to 5 ml. of formula to a piece of plastic tubing. Hold the tube up beside the bird, the tube end even with the middle of the chest. Make a mark on the tube even with the beak. The mark will act as a guide.

Hold the syringe in your right hand. The bird's body must be steadied by an assistant while you cup the bird's head in your left hand. Force the beak open slightly with the tips of your fingers, tip the head and beak slightly upward, and insert the tube. Direct the tube toward the back of the mouth, down the throat, and into the stomach area. Slowly squeeze the material in the syringe into the bird's stomach, and then gently withdraw the tube.

It is easier to pass the tube in birds than in mammals. Even adult long-necked birds such as herons are not difficult to feed; they merely require longer tubes.

While stomach-tube feeding is effective nutritionally, it should be used only as a temporary measure, when nothing else works, and only until one of the other forms of feeding can be substituted. If a bird is to get well and be self-sufficient, it must learn to feed itself.

FORCE-FEEDING SOLID FOODS

Young birds that don't yet know how to eat and injured adult birds that refuse to eat must be force-fed until they can eat on their own. We force-feed solid food more frequently than we use stomach-tube feeding, but this too is only a temporary measure.

For young birds, feed bits of cat chow moistened in formula or water. Grasp the head of the bird gently with your left hand. Pry the beak open with the fingers of your right hand.

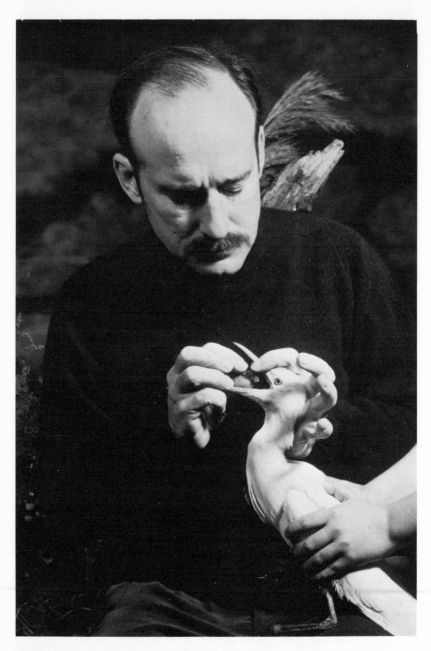

Author force-feeding canned dog food to cattle egret.

Hold the mouth open with one finger of the right hand as you place the pellet of food in the back part of the throat. Use a finger to push the pellet well down into the throat, so the bird doesn't spit it out.

Try to be firm, quick, and gentle in force-feeding so that your patient doesn't exhaust itself further by resisting your efforts.

To force-feed larger birds, offer foods they would normally be eating. An insect-eating bird can be given several crickets or several earthworms (obtained from a fishbait store).

A fish-eating heron or egret can be force-fed small bait fish (obtained from bait store). If none of these is available, try a pellet of canned dog food or several pieces of moistened dry dog food.

For long-necked birds, such as herons and egrets, the pellet may be the size and shape of a pecan or walnut. After you have placed the pellet in the back part of the throat and poked it well down into the neck with your finger, you must go one step further. Hold the beak or head in your left hand, so you don't get pecked. Then with your right hand gently feel the bird's neck till you locate the pellet of food. Push it downward along the esophagus, and on down into the chest, where it will be only a short distance from the stomach. Unless this is done, the bird will regurgitate the pellet.

Caution: When working with sharp-beaked birds such as herons and egrets, be careful. They can stab quickly with their sharp beaks. Be sure to protect your eyes. Wear protective glasses, or gently hold onto the beak to restrain the bird.

Bites or stabs elsewhere may sting but won't do you any real damage.

Force-Feeding Hawks and Owls

In force-feeding hawks and owls you must also exercise care. You will have to change your technique a little to avoid

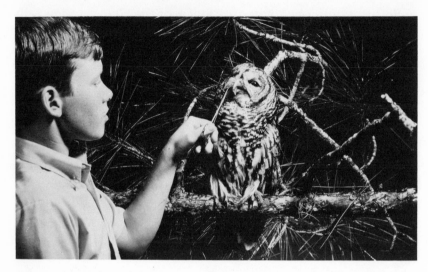

Beef heart held with forceps is offered to an injured adult barred owl.

their sharp claws and beaks. If any bird of prey grasps your hand or wrist with its talons, you must resist the temptation to shake it off. The tendon arrangement in the feet and legs of these birds only makes the sharp, curved claws penetrate more deeply if you struggle. Have a friend grasp the toes of the bird and loosen the claws, or do so yourself with your free hand. Until you know the bird, take care to avoid its claws and beak.

Feed smaller birds of prey by offering pieces of beef heart in a blunt forceps. That way your fingers don't get close to the beak. Forceps can be purchased at any drugstore.

A bird the size of a small screech owl or kestrel should be offered two or three pieces of beef heart at a feeding, each about the size of a small lima bean. Hold a piece of meat in the forceps, and touch it to the beak or to the sensitive guard hairs that owls have around their beaks. Many birds will respond by biting at whatever is touching them. When they grasp and bite at the piece of meat, release the forceps and let them have it. Most birds will hold it in their beak for fifteen to thirty seconds and then drop it.

Some hold it for a few seconds, realize it is food, and swallow it. Regardless of whether it is dropped or eaten, repeat the procedure several times until they do finally swallow.

Adult birds are taught to eat this way when they have been brought in for treatment or repair of fractures.

You will have to force-feed those that refuse to eat, by using a modification of the same technique. Place a small piece of meat in the forceps and place the forceps under the tip of the upper beak. Lift upward, and the beak will open. Without losing the upward leverage on the beak, insert the forceps into the back part of the throat and release the meat. Most birds will swallow immediately. If the bird pulls its head away from you, place your free hand behind its head, close but not touching, and try again. If it tries to move its head away from the forceps, your hand will keep it from pulling away. The activity with the forceps is distracting enough so that even adult birds seem to ignore the hand behind them.

After force-feeding several pieces of meat to a hawk or owl, allow the bird to rest for thirty minutes to an hour, then offer more. After each feeding place additional strips or pieces of meat near the bird's perch. When it starts eating on its own, start dusting the beef heart with the calcium-vitamin-mineral supplement as described previously and discontinue force-feeding.

Hawks may eat several times during the day, but fledgling or adult owls eat primarily in the evening or at night. Put four or five strips of the prepared beef heart on the perch next to an owl at dusk, and usually by morning it will have eaten them. After three or four nights you will know how much it will eat.

Some older fledglings may not eat for two or three nights. If they don't eat by the third night, force-feed them small pieces of heart with a forceps. Once an owl or hawk starts eating, it will usually eat readily from then on.

DIETARY SUPPLEMENTS
AND CALCIUM DEFICIENCIES

It is not necessary to feed your bird cod-liver oil or any other vitamin supplement. The only time any supplement is used in any of our diets is when beef heart is being fed. This meat is not adequately balanced.

All raw meat contains insufficient calcium in relation to its phosphorus content. Beef heart, for example, has a ratio of one part calcium to forty parts phosphorus. A calcium-containing powder must be added to the meat to obtain a reasonable balance, since all birds require calcium and phosphorus for building strong, healthy bones and bodies. These minerals must be given in the ratio of 1.2 parts calcium to 1 part phosphorus.

Calcium can be obtained in many forms. Most drugstores sell crushed oystershell or calcium carbonate powder, which is an excellent source of calcium. Mix the crushed tablets or calcium carbonate powder with an equal amount of a good veterinary vitamin-mineral supplement. Dusted on the heart meat, it will increase the calcium level of the diet considerably and balance the diet for feeding a hawk or owl. Use about a teaspoonful of the supplement per ounce of meat.

If calcium carbonate powder or powdered oystershell is not available, use finely crushed eggshells. Spread or dust them over the strip of meat just as you would the vitamin-mineral supplement.

Recently, deaths of seed-eating zoo birds have been traced to a calcium deficiency that resulted from eating an exclusive diet of sunflower seeds. If you are feeding your bird or animal sunflower seeds, and it refuses to eat other foods, take away almost all the sunflower seeds until it is eating other foods. Do this with any food it wants to eat exclusively. Feed fresh, leafy green vegetables such as celery and lettuce, carrots, and fruits such as peaches, grapes, oranges, bananas, and apples. Try to offer a diet as close to what the orphan will find in the wild as is practical. If birds and animals are fed a variety of foods, they are more likely to get the vitamins and minerals they need.

The general appearance and activity of any bird or animal is the best guide to whether your diet is adequate. If it eats well, has sleek, shiny feathers, flies well, and is strong and vigorous, you are feeding an adequate diet. If the feathers are poor and the bird is weak, consult your veterinarian for help.

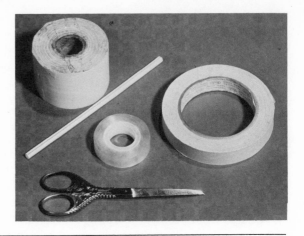

8

First Aid for All Birds

WHICH BIRDS NEED FIRST AID?

A bird with a leg dangling loose and limp as it hops across the lawn, or with a wing dropping awkwardly at its side, or a bird with an open wound obviously needs help. A bird sitting at the edge of the road in the face of passing traffic, a bird huddled on the sidewalk in the rain rather than taking refuge in a tree, a bird falling each time it tries to hop or fly; all of these birds are in need of help. Not quite so apparent, however, and just as much in need of help is the bird with eyes closed sitting on the ground, resting its head on its shoulders, its feathers all fluffed up. The condition of this bird would be more obvious if other birds of the same species were flying around it, sleek, bright, and chipper, while it sat with the "droops."

Before you attempt to approach or pick up such a bird, study its behavior. Watch it for a while. Try to determine what is abnormal about the bird. Is its leg hurt? Its wing? If so, which one? Can it fly at all? Does it fall if it tries to run? A study of the bird will indicate where and what the problem is. This will not be so apparent once you get it home. For once it is confined to a cage, chances are it won't move.

Do not take the bird home if you don't feel you can help. If you don't think you'll be able to splint a leg or wing or clean up a wound, leave the bird where it is. If the bird can eat and can hop about even awkwardly, it will probably be all right and should be left alone.

If, however, you feel the bird needs help, and if you can find or provide the help that is needed, approach slowly and use the minimum amount of force necessary to capture the bird.

You should keep in mind, if you decide to start treating a weak, injured, or sick bird, that you may not be able to save it. It is sometimes better for an injured creature to die without pain than to spend the rest of its life deformed and caged. At such times, euthanasia, which is a painless death to prevent suffering, may be the best and most humane solution for certain injured animals or birds. To have tried to help a less fortunate creature is what is important. Those that you do save make up for the personal hurt that occurs when a creature must be euthanized.

APPROACHING AN INJURED BIRD

Never chase a bird. Sick birds and injured birds will often die from the extra stress of rough handling or chasing, so patience and gentleness are important.

Very young birds seem to respond quite well when you approach slowly, talk quietly, and handle them gently. However, older birds do not like to be handled. It is better to herd them gently into a corner or even a cardboard box. Approach quietly and cover them gently with your jacket or shirt, which can be tucked around them and used to carry them when nothing else is available. When they are covered and cannot see you, they are much less fearful.

You can most effectively capture injured hawks and owls by herding them into a cardboard box lying on its side. The box seems to represent security to these birds, and many will enter the box with very little herding. Fold in the flaps to confine it and transport the bird to where the necessary aid can be given.

BASIC CARE

Basic nursing care is the same for all birds in need of first aid. It consists of providing warmth, security, water, and food.

Warmth is very important. An adult bird does not need extra warmth under normal circumstances. But it is very much in need of extra warmth if it is sick or has been injured. Warmth is as important as food or medication if your patient is to survive. Provide warmth from a 100-watt light bulb. For an adult bird, suspend the bulb nearby as it rests on a perch or on the floor of the cage.

Select a cage according to the size of the bird. Generally, it should be at least $30'' \times 30'' \times 36''$. Use a smaller cage when you wish to restrict the movement of a severely injured bird.

Often warmth and temporary security are all a bird needs to recover. Do not handle it any more than is absolutely necessary. If it begins to move about normally, without falling or losing its balance, release it.

If a bird is to be kept for additional care or treatment, offer it fresh water and a variety of foods. Some birds are seed eaters; other eat insects or fruits. You must know something about your patient to provide the proper choice of foods. Read about your patient in one of the good bird books. Then offer those foods that it is most likely to be familiar with. When in doubt, offer a wide variety of foods to see what it will eat.

CHILLED BIRDS

Birds may be found wet and chilled after several days of continuous cold rain. Birds that migrate north before much food is available are particularly susceptible. You may find them sitting wet and bedraggled on the ground or on a low limb. Weak from lack of food, they become much more susceptible to chilling.

Once a bird's feathers get wet, they lose their insulation value. The bird becomes chilled rapidly. Such a bird will not resist being picked up. You can easily capture it and carry it inside.

Suspend a 100-watt bulb near a perch in a cage to provide heat to dry the feathers. After the bird is warm and its feathers are thoroughly dry and fluffy, offer it food, and then release it. Since it is wild and may hurt itself by flying into the sides of the cage in an attempt to escape, keep it no longer than necessary.

CONCUSSION-TYPE INJURIES

Sometimes a bird becomes confused and flies into a solid object, hitting its head. This results in concussion. You may find such a bird lying unconscious beside a building. As long as it is still alive, it has a chance. Pick up the bird, bring it indoors, and provide it with warmth and shelter. Surprisingly, after a few hours of rest many of these birds will be completely recovered and can be released. Others, however, recover more slowly and may need several days of rest before they can be released.

A bird suffering from a concussion may remain unconscious for a day or longer. Place this bird in a nest box prepared as for a baby altricial bird, supporting it in a normal, comfortably, semiupright position. Position a thermometer close to the resting bird, and position a light bulb to provide a constant temperature of 85° F.

On the second day, if the bird is not moving about, offer a tiny bird food by the toothpick formula technique, discussed in the previous chapter, and offer a larger bird formula with a medicine dropper.

If a bird is severely injured, it may take a week or longer for your patient to recover. Provide clean, fresh water and food for it and handle it only when absolutely necessary. When it begins to hop about normally, without falling or losing its balance, it is ready to be released. Release the bird in a place where you can recapture it easily in case it cannot fly well.

INTESTINAL INFECTION

The most common bacterial disease is intestinal infection. Normal bird droppings consist of thick black material from the intestinal tract combined with a white paste-like kidney excretion. When the black material becomes soft and light in color, this usually signals the start of an intestinal upset or infection. If allowed to progress, the droppings become watery, light-colored, and foamy in appearance. If this situation develops with an orphan you are raising, or if the droppings are loose in an adult, start administering antibiotic at once.

Antibiotics

Tetracycline, the same antibiotic recommended for mammals, is used for birds as well. You can obtain it from a veterinarian or the pharmacist by prescription.

The amount of antibiotic to use depends on the size of the bird. A bird the size of a screech owl or a blue jay would normally receive a total daily dose of 15 to 20 mg. One 250-mg. capsule contains enough antibiotic to treat a bird this size for about two weeks.

If you wish to be exact, weigh the bird on a postal scale and calculate the correct dosage. Use a figure of 4 mg. of antibiotic per ounce of the bird's weight per day, divided into three to four doses.

A less exacting way would be to place the tiniest pinch of antibiotic on a piece of moistened cat chow at each feeding, four times a day. If you remember the amount in the capsule is enough for at least fifty doses for a bird the size of the average blue jay or screech owl, you will realize what is meant by a tiny pinch. Resist the temptation to give more than the smallest amount. If necessary, actually divide the capsules into fifteen separate piles on a piece of wax paper. Each little pile then represents one day's total dosage.

PROBLEM EATER

Your bird patient may not want to eat. If it is running a fever, badly frightened, very weak, or just not familiar with the food offered, the bird usually won't want to eat.

If you are giving medication such as antibiotics, the bird must be force-fed frequently enough during the day to get the required medication into it. The cat chow moistened and softened with the milk and egg formula is usually used for force-feeding. The required antibiotic is placed on the bite-sized bit of moistened cat chow and force-fed.

Offer a variety of foods, fruits, and seeds in the hope you can find something to tempt the bird's appetite. In addition, provide good nursing care of warmth, a secure cage, and fresh water.

OIL-CONTAMINATED BIRDS

Oil spills don't occur only on ocean beaches. A bird may become coated with oil from contact with waste oil and with contaminated inland water as well. The oil does damage to the birds in several ways. It mats the feathers together so that they lose their insulation value. The bird then chills, becomes lethargic, and, if the outside temperature is cold, dies of exposure. Or else the bird preens itself and, as it does so, ingests the oil. Among other things this causes damage to its intestinal lining. The intestine can no longer absorb water properly, and the bird often dies of dehydration.

Although the oil spill problem is not a new one, public concern over its effects on wildlife is fairly recent. Techniques in caring for oil-contaminated birds are changing from day to day, and there are no pat answers.

The actual procedure for cleaning a group of oiled birds is a complex one, requiring expensive equipment and materials which may be inflammable. The solvents used are very difficult for the general public to obtain. Therefore, the best action you can take if you find an oil spill involving a large number of birds is to evaluate the situation and seek professional help. Try to determine how many birds are involved. Is the oil a heavy, thick, tarry substance or a thin, volatile oil similar to gasoline? How large an area does the spill cover? When you have as much information as you can gather, report the spill to the nearest Coast Guard station or Environmental Protection Agency office. Also contact the local Audubon Society for volunteers to pick up the birds. Most states have an oil spill plan involving the Coast Guard, game and fish departments, veterinary associations, and wildlife groups. If the spill is serious and involves much wildlife, a professional cleaning team will be sent to the area as well as specialized equipment to clean up the spill itself.

You may collect the contaminated birds and place them in cardboard boxes while waiting for help to arrive. For holding all but the largest of birds, cardboard file boxes 10″ × 12″ × 14″ are satisfactory. Partially fill the boxes with shredded newspaper or other soft bedding. Normally, no more than one bird should be placed in the box. If the birds are quite small, however, two or more of the same species may be placed in the same box. The boxes should have lids in order to create darkness. This will keep the birds quiet and keep them from preening. The birds should be shielded in cool weather to prevent their chilling and in warm weather to prevent heat prostration.

There will be many opportunities for you to assist when the cleaning team moves in to treat the contaminated wildlife.

You may clean them yourself if only one or two birds are found and help is not available. Two people are needed for this procedure.

The safest thing for you to use to clean the birds is mineral oil, which may be obtained at any drugstore. It should be warmed to 100° F. Pour about 2 inches of warm mineral oil into a plastic dishpan. Gently place the contaminated bird in the oil. One person should gently restrain the bird as it stands in a normal upright position while the other does the actual cleaning.

If the bird has been contaminated with a thin oil, such as gasoline, diesel fuel, or waste motor oil, scoop up the mineral oil in your cupped hand and trickle it over the bird wherever the contaminating oil exists. Gently separate the feathers with your hand so the oil penetrates and dilutes the contaminating oil.

If the contaminating oil is a heavy, tarry oil, the warm mineral oil is trickled over the contaminating masses, softening them and dissolving them away. Gently massaging the tarry blobs with your free hand will speed up the softening process.

Discard the mineral oil in the dishpan when it becomes dirty in either cleaning procedure. Place the same amount of clean, warm mineral oil in the dishpan and repeat the cleaning procedure until the oil in the dishpan no longer becomes dirty. A moderately contaminated bird may require two gallons or more of mineral oil to get it clean.

With soft rags, blot the excess mineral oil from the feathers after the bird is clean. When you have finished, the bird will preen itself, removing the balance of the mineral oil over the next several days. The mineral oil is inert and not harmful if it is swallowed by the bird.

The bird must be kept warm for the next several days, since the oily feathers are not good insulators against the cold. Provide the basic nursing care of shelter, warmth, and food, until the plumage is completely back to normal. Then the bird should be freed.

Remember that migratory water birds are protected by federal law. You must have permission to keep one, even for treatment. Notify the local wildlife officer of the number and type of birds you have, and how long you estimate they will be in your care. They will tell you how to obtain whatever additional permission you may need to hold the birds for treatment.

FRACTURES

In any fracture, if you aren't sure how to proceed, take the bird to a veterinarian. If there is no veterinarian available to help you, try gently and carefully to help the bird.

A broken leg is a common injury. It is usually not critical to a bird's survival but, of course, should be repaired if possible. Most of these procedures require two people.

Lower Leg

If the lower part of the fractured leg is still warm, indicating good circulation, healing will probably occur if the leg is properly immobilized. To do this, make a splint and tape it in place.

FOR SMALL BIRDS. For small birds, such as a sparrow, mockingbird, blue jay, or robin, use a large plastic soda straw.

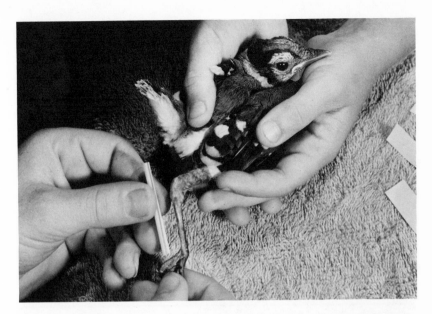

Flattened plastic straw, cut to length, and bent into V shape along its length, is applied to lower leg fracture and taped in place.

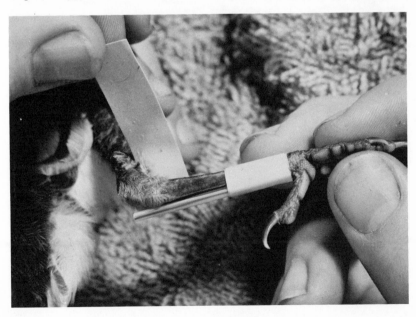

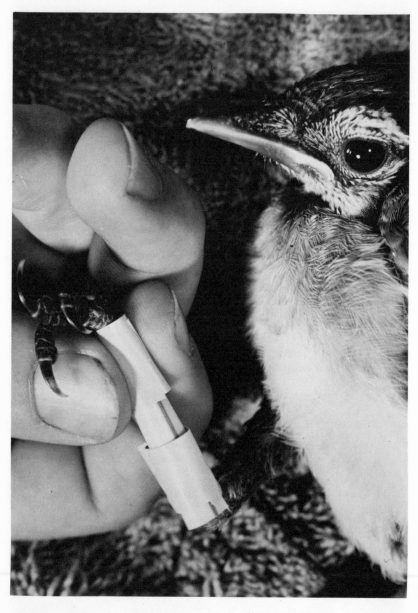

Let the splint remain in place until it wears off or the bird removes it.

Cut a piece of straw about the same length as the broken bone. Flatten it, then fold it double along its length and bend it into a V shape. Place the injured leg in the V trough of the straw and tape it gently in place with Scotch or Dermalite (Johnson & Johnson). Let the splint remain in place until it wears off or the bird removes it. By that time the leg should be well healed. If the splint comes partially loose and is dangling, remove the rest.

FOR LARGER BIRDS. For larger birds, such as pheasants, owls, hawks, ducks, or egrets, plastic splint material, such as strips cut from a gallon plastic milk jug, is especially good, because it is light, strong, and does not absorb water. The splint material must be as long as the bone to be repaired and rigid enough to support the bone while it heals. Place a thin piece of plastic or rubber foam padding between the splint and the leg. Tape the splint snugly, but not tightly, along the full length of the fractured bone. If the fracture is close to a joint, extend your splint and tape across the joint for additional support. Applied properly, a splint allows the leg almost normal movement.

Upper Leg

This requires two people. Have someone hold the bird while you tape the leg. Use Dermalite tape if you can. Dermalite tape does not damage the feathers as much as Scotch tape or adhesive tapes. Also, it is waterproof, lightweight, easily cut and applied, and sticks well.

In a fracture of the upper leg, tape the leg against the body in a normal position and allow it to remain taped for three weeks, if possible. Three weeks is ideal, but many birds manage to rip the tape off within two weeks. However, if you allow them two more weeks of rest in the cage before permitting them to fly, they will usually be healed.

Be sure the tape is not so tight around the chest that it

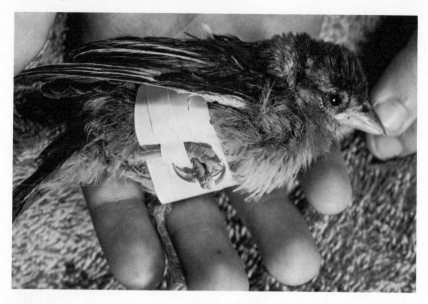

Tape wrapped around body and leg immobilizes bone ends in upper leg fractures.

restricts breathing. Be sure, also, not to obstruct the vent, the opening from which fecal material is evacuated.

AMPUTATION. If the fractured portion of the leg is cold and clammy, it indicates that circulation has been severely damaged. When the break area is badly mutilated and dirty, the fractured bones often will not heal. These must be amputated. Your veterinarian will help you or will do it for you. The nerves have probably also been damaged, so pain is not severe. Amputated legs generally heal well, and birds can manage well with one leg.

Fractured Wings

These, too, are common injuries in birds. Repairing fractured wings usually takes two people. Restrain the bird gently, to avoid further damage to circulation in the fractured wing. If the fractured part is as warm as the other parts of the

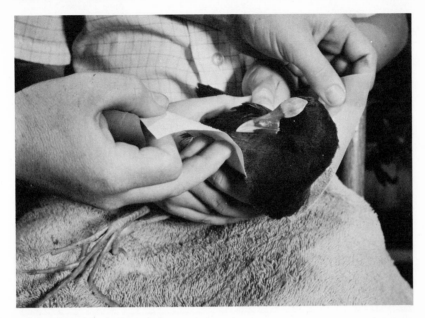

Tape applied to hold injured wing in place. The other wing must be kept free so that the bird can maintain its balance.

bird's body, then circulation is still satisfactory and the wing will usually heal.

For small birds use your fingertips to place the bone ends in position while an assistant holds the bird for you. With Dermalite tape, tape the bird's wing folded against its body in its normal resting position. Tape only the fractured wing. Allowing the other wing to be free will help the bird to balance itself. Allow the wing to remain taped for three weeks.

Open Wound or Compound Fracture

Give an antibiotic for seven to ten days in order to prevent infection to a bird with an open wound or a compound fracture. Administer the antibiotic in the bird's food, as described in the section on intestinal infection.

If the flesh is torn and bone ends are exposed, the treatment is more complicated and proper veterinary care is more essential. Where such help is not available, clean the wound and bone ends with a mild antiseptic such as Zephiran, which can be obtained at a drugstore. After cleaning, place the bones in their normal position with the fractured ends touching and apply an antibiotic powder to the open wound. Then tape the wing folded against the body in the normal resting position.

Here, too, apply the tape just tightly enough to hold the bones in position but not so tightly that it will interfere with breathing.

Fractures in Large Birds

Larger birds, such as herons, egrets, hawks, and owls, usually require professional veterinary care if the birds are to fly again when they recover from a fractured wing. Allow your veterinarian to examine the bird and suggest proper treatment. If he can repair the broken wing, you will still have to provide nursing care if the bird is to survive.

If the wing is not repairable or circulation has been severely damaged, a part of the wing may have to be amputated. If even a portion of a wing has been amputated, the bird will never fly again. Unless you are prepared to take care of the bird for the rest of its life or know of a wildlife sanctuary, zoo, or other place where the bird can receive permanent care, it is probably more humane to let your veterinarian euthanize it than to keep it in a cage for the rest of its life.

Most adult birds accept minimal handling without resentment. Mature, grown birds never become friendly, but they will accept being carried on your hand, being stroked on the head and chest, and will learn not to try to escape when you approach.

When its injury has healed and the bird is able to fly, release it in the area where it was found. If you are doubtful about its ability to fly, and you have space around your home, you may release it there. In this way you can recapture it if necessary, or feed it conveniently until it is completely rehabilitated.

Your patient will usually stay where you release it for several hours or longer. If the bone breaks when it attempts to fly, you must start all over again.

If the bird takes off and flies successfully, you have the deep satisfaction of knowing you have given it another chance at life.

Afterword

Many of the techniques used in this book have been adapted from established techniques in the field of veterinary medicine. Information from colleagues, clients, and veterinary journals, such as the journal of the American Association of Zoo Veterinarians, contributed part of the framework to build upon. Additional information was gleaned from the trials and errors of our personal experiences in raising wild babies.

This book is not meant to be the final work on the raising of wild orphans. Rather it is the first step in the organization and accumulation of knowledge in handling native wild babies.

I have purposely not spoken of seabirds. We live inland in Florida and our experiences with these species have been limited to the care of a few injured gulls.

I would welcome suggestions and comments from people who read this book and use it, and from those engaged in similar endeavors.

W. J. WEBER D.V.M.

Migratory Birds

Game Migratory Birds

Anatidae—Wild ducks, geese, brant, and swans
Charadriidae—Plovers, turnstones, killdeer, and surfbirds
Columbidae—Wild doves and pigeons
Gruidae—Little brown, sandhill, and whooping cranes
Haematopodidae—Oyster catchers
Phalaropodidae—Phalaropes
Rallidae—Rails, soras, coots, and gallinules
Recurvirostridae—Avocets and stilts
Scolopacidae—Sandpipers, curlews, yellowlegs, knots, dowitchers, god-
    wits, willets, woodcock, snipe, and sanderlings

Non-Game Migratory Birds

Alaudidae—Horned larks
Alcidae—Auks, auklets, murres, murrelets, puffins, guillemots, and
    dovekies
Apodidae—Micropodidae, and swifts
Ardeidae—Herons, bitterns, and egrets

143

Bombycillidae—Waxwings

Caprimulgidae—Whippoorwills, poorwills, nighthawks, chuck-will's-widows, and pauraques

Certhiidae—Brown creepers

Cuculidae—Cuckoos, anis, and roadrunners

Fringillidae—Cardinals, grosbeaks, buntings, finches, sparrows, towhees, juncos, crossbills, dickcissels, and longspurs

Gaviidae—Loons

Hirundinidae—Swallows and martins

Hydrobatidae—Petrels

Icteridae—Bobolinks, meadowlarks, orioles, grackles, blackbirds, and cowbirds

Laniidae—Shrikes

Laridae—Gulls, terns, and kittiwakes

Mimidae—Mockingbirds, catbirds, and thrashers

Motacillidae—Pipits and wagtails

Paridae—Titmice, chickadees, bushtits, and verdins

Parulidae—Warblers, ovenbirds, water thrushes, chats, and redstarts

Picidae—Woodpeckers, flickers, and sapsuckers

Podicipedidae—Grebes

Procellariidae—Shearwaters and fulmars

Ptilogonatidae—Phainopeplas

Sittidae—Nuthatches

Stercorariidae—Skuas and jaegers

Sulidae—Gannets and boobies

Sylviidae—Kinglets and gnatcatchers

Thraupidae—Tanagers

Trochilidae—Hummingbirds

Troglodytidae—Wrens

Turdidae—Robins, thrushes, bluebirds, solitaires, and wheatears

Tyrannidae—Tyrant flycatchers, kingbirds, peewees, and phoebes

Vireonidae—Vireos

Regional Offices of Fish and Wildlife Service

Mailing Address: Regional Director
                   Bureau of Sport Fisheries and Wildlife
                   (Refer to the lists below for the balance
                   of address that serves your state)

Region 1:   P.O. Box 3737, Portland, Oregon   97208
            234-4050 (Area Code) 503

Region 2:   P.O. Box 1306, Albuquerque, New Mexico   87103
            766-2321 (Area Code) 505

Region 3:   Federal Building, Fort Snelling, Twin Cities,
            Minnesota   55111   725-3500 (Area Code) 612

Region 4:   17 Executive Park Drive, N.E., Atlanta, Georgia   30329
            526-4675 (Area Code) 404

Region 5:   U.S. Post Office and Courthouse, Boston,
            Massachusetts   02109   223-2961 (Area Code) 607

Region 6:   P.O. Box 25486, Denver Federal Center, Denver,
            Colorado   80225   234-2209 (Area Code) 303

Alaska Area: 813 D Street, Anchorage, Alaska   99501
               8-206-583-0150 (Seattle)
               Ask for: 907-165-4864

Rare and Endangered Species

Since 1844, when the great auk disappeared from North America, followed by the Carolina parakeet, the passenger pigeon, the heath hen, and the Labrador duck, some seventy-eight species and forty-nine sub-species have become extinct over the world. The fact that a North American and a World Endangered Species list has been prepared and will be kept up to date demonstrates that governments are becoming concerned over this rapid loss of animal populations. The fact that a species appears on this list does nothing to ensure its survival. For unfortunately, that is all it is—a list. It is up to individual states that have an endangered species within their borders to initiate the measures which will enable these creatures to survive.

Following is the list prepared by the United States Department of the Interior.

Rare and Endangered Mammals

Indiana Bat (E)
Spotted Bat (R)
Utah Prairie Dog (E)

Kaibab Squirrel (R)
Delmarva Peninsula Fox Squirrel (E)

Block Island Meadow Vole (R)
Beach Meadow Vole (R)
Whales:
  Gray Whale (R)
  Blue Whale (E)
  Humpback Whale (E)
  Atlantic Right Whale (E)
  Pacific Right Whale (E)
  Bowhead Whale (R)
Eastern Timber Wolf (E)
Texas Red Wolf (E)
San Joaquin Kit Fox (E)
Glacier Bear (R)
Grizzly Bear (R)
Black-Footed Ferret (E)
Southern Sea Otter (R)
Florida Panther (E)
Ribbon Seal (R)
Caribbean Monk Seal (E)
Hawaiian Monk Seal (R)
Guadalupe Fur Seal (E)
Florida Manatee or Florida Sea
  Cow (E)
Tule Elk or Dwarf Elk (R)
Key Deer (E)
Columbian White-tailed Deer (E)
Sonoran Pronghorn (E)
California Bighorn (R)
Peninsular Bighorn (R)

Rare and Endangered Birds

Newell's Manx Shearwater (R)
Hawaiian Dark-rumped Petrel (E)
California Least Tern (E)
Florida Great White Heron (R)
Nene (Hawaiian Goose) (E)
Aleutian Canada Goose (E)
Tule White-fronted Goose (E)
Laysan Duck (E)
Hawaiian Duck (Koloa) (E)

Mexican Duck (E)
California Condor (E)
Florida Everglade Kite (Florida
  Snail Kite) (E)
Hawaiian Hawk (Io) (E)
Short-tailed Hawk (R)
Southern Bald Eagle (E)
Prairie Falcon (R)
American Peregrine Falcon (E)
Northern Greater Prairie Chicken
  (R)
Attwater's Greater Prairie
  Chicken (E)
Lesser Prairie Chicken (R)
Masked Bobwhite (E)
Whooping Crane (E)
Greater Sandhill Crane (R)
Florida Sandhill Crane (R)
Yuma Clapper Rail (E)
California Clapper Rail (R)
Light-footed Clapper Rail (E)
California Black Rail (R)
Hawaiian Gallinule (E)
Hawaiian Coot (E)
Eskimo Curlew (E)
Hawaiian Stilt (E)
Puerto Rican Plain Pigeon (E)
Puerto Rican Parrot (E)
Puerto Rican Whip-Poor-Will (R)
American Ivory-billed Wood-
  pecker (E)
Northern Red-cockaded Wood-
  pecker (E)
Southern Red-cockaded Wood-
  pecker (E)
Hawaiian Crow (Alala) (E)
Puaiohi (Small Kauai Thrush)
  (E)
Large Kauai Thrush (R)
Nihoa Millerbird (E)
Kauai Oo (Oo Aa) (E)

Crested Honeycreeper
(Akohekohe) (E)
Molokai Creeper (Kakawahie)
(E)
Akiapolaau (E)
Kauai Akialoa (E)
Kauai Nukupuu (E)
Maui Nukupuu (E)
Laysan Finch (E)
Nihoa Finch (E)
Ou (E)
Palila (E)
Maui Parrotbill (E)
Bachman's Warbler (E)
Golden-cheeked Warbler (R)
Kirtland's Warbler (E)
Ipswich Sparrow (R)
Dusky Seaside Sparrow (E)
Cape Sable Sparrow (E)

Rare and Endangered Reptiles

Bog Turtle (R)
American Alligator (E)
Blunt-nosed Leopard Lizard (E)
San Francisco Garter Snake (E)
Puerto Rican Boa (E)

**Rare and Endangered
Amphibians**

Santa Cruz Long-toed Sala-
mander (E)
Texas Blind Salamander (E)
Limestone Salamander (R)
Black Toad, Inyo County Toad
(R)
Houston Toad (E)
Pine Barrens Tree Frog (R)
Vegas Valley Leopard Frog (R)

Composition of Animal Milks by Percentage

	Solids	Fat	Protein	Carbo-hydrates
Cow (*Bovidae*)	11.9	3.5	3.0	4.6
Dog (*Canidae*)	24.0	10.5	7.9	3.8
Cat (*Felidae*)	20.0	6.5	9.0	6.8
Rabbit (*Leporidae*)	30.5	10.4	15.5	1.9
Mouse (*Muridae*)	25.8	12.1	9.0	3.2
Pig (*Suidae*)	20.0	7.3	6.6	5.0
Sheep (*Bovidae*)	20.5	8.6	5.7	5.4
Goat (*Bovidae*)	12.8	4.1	3.7	4.2
Opossum (*Didelphidae*)	14.0	4.7	4.0	4.5
Gray Squirrel (*Sciuridae*)	26.6	12.6	9.2	3.4
Beaver (*Castoridae*)	33.0	19.8	9.0	2.2
Coyote (*Canidae*)	24.5	10.7	9.9	2.3
Fox (*Canidae*)	18.1	6.3	6.2	4.6
Raccoon (*Procyonidae*)	13.4	3.9	4.0	4.7
Otter (*Mustelidae*)	35.9	23.9	11.0	.1

Deer (*Cervidae*)	23.1	8.0	10.6	2.8
Pronghorn Antelope				
(*Antilocapridae*)	25.2	13.0	6.9	4.0

This information courtesy of Borden, Inc.

Suggested for Further Reading

1. Cahalane, Victor. *Mammals of North America.* New York, The Macmillan Company, 1961.
   An excellent book on mammals, the best I have read.

2. *Wild Animals of North America.* Washington, D.C., National Geographic Society, 1960.
   A good book with general information on animals.

3. Allen, Arthur A. *Stalking Birds with Color Camera.* Washington, D.C., National Geographic Society, 1963.
   This is more than a photography book. Dr. Allen gives a great deal of background to help the reader understand and work with birds.

4. Pettengill, Olin, Jr. *Ornithology in Laboratory and Field.* Minneapolis, Burgess, 1970.
   A study text on birds for post-high school students.

5. Robbins, C. S., Brunn, B., and Zim, H. S. *Birds of North America.* New York, Golden Press, 1966.
   The easiest to use of the identification guides.

6. Wetmore, Alex. *Song and Garden Birds of North America.* Washington, D.C., National Geographic Society, 1964.
   Identification and interesting facts about the songbirds.

7. Wetmore, Alex. *Water, Prey, and Game Birds of North America.* Washington, D.C., National Geographic Society, 1965.
   General background for understanding this group of birds.

Index